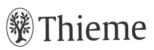

Muscle Function Testing—
A Visual Guide

Karin Wieben
Physical Therapist
Timmendorfer Strand, Germany

Bernd Falkenberg
Physical Therapist
Iserlohn, Germany

191 illustrations

Thieme
Stuttgart · New York · Delhi · Rio de Janeiro

Library of Congress Cataloging-in-Publication Data

Wieben, Karin, author.
  [Muskelfunktion. English]
  Muscle function testing : a visual guide /
Karin Wieben, Bernd Falkenberg.
    p. ; cm.
  "This book is an authorized translation of the
6th German edition published and copyrighted
2012 by Georg Thieme Verlag, Stuttgart. Title of
the German edition: Muskelfunktion: Prüfung
und klinische Bedeutung."
  Includes bibliographical references and index.
  ISBN 978-3-13-199721-0 (alk. paper) –
  ISBN 978-3-13-199731-9 (ebook)
  I. Falkenberg, Bernd, author. II. Title.
  [DNLM: 1. Muscle Diseases–diagnosis.
2. Muscles–physiology. 3. Musculoskeletal
Physiological Phenomena. WE 500]
  RC925.7
  616.7'4075–dc23   2015006174

This book is an authorized translation of the 6th
German edition published and copyrighted 2012 by
Georg Thieme Verlag, Stuttgart. Title of the German
edition: Muskelfunktion: Prüfung und klinische Bedeutung

Translator: Dr. phil. Karen Leube,
Leube Translation and Language Services,
Aachen, Germany

Drawings: Rose Baumann, Schriesheim;
Helmut Holtermann, Dannenberg
Illustrations: M. Voll and K. Wesker
Anatomic watercolors taken from Schünke
et al. Prometheus. Lernatlas der Anatomie.
Kopf und Neuroanatomie

© 2015 Georg Thieme Verlag KG
Thieme Publishers Stuttgart
Rüdigerstrasse 14, 70469 Stuttgart,
Germany, +49 [0]711 8931 421
customerservice@thieme.de

Thieme Publishers New York
333 Seventh Avenue, New York, NY 10001, USA,
1-800-782-3488
customerservice@thieme.com

Thieme Publishers Delhi
A-12, second floor, Sector-2, Noida-201301,
Uttar Pradesh, India, +91 120 45 566 00
customerservice@thieme.in

Thieme Publishers Rio
Thieme Publicações Ltda.
Argentina Building, 16th floor, Ala A,
228 Praia do Botafogo,
Rio de Janeiro 22250-040 Brazil,
+55 21 3736–3631

Cover design: Thieme Publishing Group
Typesetting by Ziegler und Müller,
Kirchentellinsfurt, Germany

Printed in Italy by L. E. G. O., Vicenza

ISBN 9783131997210

Also available as an e-book:
eISBN 9783131997319

Important note: Medicine is an everchanging sci-
ence undergoing continual development. Research
and clinical experience are continually expanding
our knowledge, in particular our knowledge of
proper treatment and drug therapy. Insofar as this
book mentions any dosage or application, readers
may rest assured that the authors, editors, and publishers have made every effort to ensure that such
references are in accordance with **the state of
knowledge at the time of production of the book.**
  Nevertheless, this does not involve, imply, or ex-
press any guarantee or responsibility on the part of
the publishers in respect to any dosage instructions
and forms of applications stated in the book. **Every
user is requested to examine carefully** the manufacturers' leaflets accompanying each drug and to
check, if necessary in consultation with a physician
or specialist, whether the dosage schedules men-
tioned therein or the contraindications stated by
the manufacturers differ from the statements made
in the present book. Such examination is particularly important with drugs that are either rarely used
or have been newly released on the market. Every
dosage schedule or every form of application used
is entirely at the user's own risk and responsibility.
The authors and publishers request every user to report to the publishers any discrepancies or inaccur-
acies noticed. If errors in this work are found after
publication, errata will be posted at www.thieme.
com on the product description page.
  Some of the product names, patents, and regis-
tered designs referred to in this book are in fact reg-
istered trademarks or proprietary names even
though specific reference to this fact is not always
made in the text. Therefore, the appearance of a
name without designation as proprietary is not to
be construed as a representation by the publisher
that it is in the public domain.

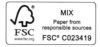

Contents

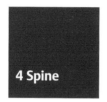

4 Spine

5 Upper Extremity

Foreword

Nearly 80 years have passed since the first attempts to evaluate muscular deficits and record comparable results were undertaken (Daniels et al. 1962). In the development of muscle testing over the years, two things stand out: the key role these procedures play in daily physical therapy routine and the efforts by users to make muscle testing even more practical and functional. The testing methods are used to determine the status quo when patients are taken on for treatment. In addition, they are useful tools for monitoring therapy results through follow-up testing at regular intervals and for determining the final diagnosis. This provides physicians, physical therapists, occupational and sports therapists with information about treatment paths and any necessary modifications, recovery from paralysis, support required for patients to manage their activities of daily living by themselves, and their treatment needs following discharge. Testing allows patients to see their treatment progress, which reduces their anxiety, while therapists can adapt treatment methods to the individually determined functional circumstances. Test results provide coaches and athletic trainers working in sports for rehabilitation and for disabled participants with access to valuable documents for evaluating athletic performance ranges. Uniform principles at the national and international level allow for comparable tests when using medical, physical therapy, or occupational therapy treatment approaches.

The range of spinal cord injury symptoms is broad and includes both complete and partial paralysis. The tests presented in this book are especially well-suited for analyzing isolated deficits and for evaluating methods for testing these deficits, as well as possible compensatory mechanisms. While, in the 1950s, peripheral paralysis in patients with polio was the driving force behind the expansion of existing test methods, for many years it has been the improved treatment methods for spinal cord injuries that have driven this process.

Karin Wieben was head of the physical therapy department of the Spinal Cord Injury Center of the BUK Hospital in Hamburg for many years, and Bernd Falkenberg was one of her team members there. Together and in close collaboration with the rest of the team they developed the concepts presented in this book, which emerged from their daily work with spinal cord injured patients, starting from the days surrounding the accident through to the completion of comprehensive rehabilitation.

They have now added an additional grade to the tried and tested, internationally recognized evaluation system comprising muscle function grades 0 to 5. Adding grade 6 permits statements to be made about the endurance of a movement, which may allow residual weakness to be identified. The authors have added the usual symptoms related to paralysis to the functional descriptions, and have also described the impact of residual weaknesses on everyday movements. This provides an additional method

for recognizing masked deficits and making therapeutic approaches accessible.

Pioneers who break new ground have to be prepared to receive both agreement and criticism. The outcome of debate is the decisive factor in whether or not new or complementary methods will enjoy broad application. No matter what, such debate offers to clarify a number of unanswered questions. This fuels progress, and there is no doubt that the material in this book will contribute to this progress.

Professor F.-W. Meinecke
Former Head of the Spinal Cord Injury
Center of the BUK Hospital
Hamburg, Germany

Preface

"Keep what works and be open to new ideas."

The German version of this book, which has been published in six editions, has been part of the medical repertoire for over 20 years. The motto above has served as a guiding principle as we revised each edition.

Since the muscle testing in its current form has proven effective, we did not feel that any conceptual modifications were necessary. However, the changes to the sixth German edition, which is the basis for this first English edition, involved technical additions that have modified the layout. The chapter on the foundations of muscle testing has been expanded to include supplementary explanations and anatomical drawings. The chapter on testing of the muscles of facial expression and mastication is completely new. We have added these topics to provide guidelines for therapists working with muscles of the face and head.

The quick tests presented here allow examiners to obtain rapid initial insight into the muscular situation of the extremities or the trunk. Later on, a detailed muscle analysis using specific muscle tests can be performed.

Scientific progress is possible only if topics are dealt with critically. We sincerely hope that this book will provide a small contribution to this process and we welcome your feedback. We look forward to engaging with and building on your comments. We are especially pleased that this book will now be accessible to therapists in the United Kingdom, where muscle testing originated, and hope that the response there will be positive.

We would like to thank Eva Gruenewald and Fritz Koller of Georg Thieme Verlag for their valuable assistance with the realization of the new edition of the German book. Our gratitude also goes to Angelika Findgott and Joanne Stead of Thieme Publishers for the production of the English version. We are especially thankful to our photographer Christian Knospe for his unending patience and his professional standards. Our thanks go to Irina Schatz, my daughter Anne Falkenberg, and my son Max Falkenberg for kindly agreeing to pose as models for the photos.

Karin Wieben, Bernd Falkenberg

1
Fundamentals

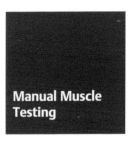

Manual Muscle Testing

With manual muscle testing, the strength of a muscle group can be determined with minimal effort by using defined muscle movements.

In patients with neurological disorders, accurate statements about muscle function are helpful for performing differential diagnosis and for locating damage. They can also provide information to support a prognosis. Furthermore, muscle testing is a valuable tool for analyzing muscular imbalances as objectively as possible. By regularly repeating these tests, objective statements can be made about the course of physical therapy. The attainment of treatment objectives can be monitored and the treatment plan can be adjusted accordingly. Although using instruments or electromyography to measure muscle strength is more objective, these methods require significantly more effort. In addition, they can measure only certain muscle groups and cannot be used in all settings.

Prerequisites for Accurate Results of Muscle Testing

To evaluate the active range of motion in a joint, the examiner must have in-depth knowledge of joint mechanics as well as the muscle's anatomy and function. For the test to be reliable, it must be carried out accurately, precisely, and rigorously. Moreover, the examiner needs to have sufficient experience to come up with an objective assessment after weighing all the criteria.

Inaccurate muscle testing can create confusion because of false results and can result in incorrect conclusions being drawn.

The following points must be observed when performing muscle testing (Janda 2009, Montgomery and Hislop 2007):

- Muscle testing must always be performed with the patient in the correct starting position, while maintaining the proper planes of motion.
- If the patient needs to be stabilized in order to perform the test, the examiner should always do this proximal to the joint being moved.
- To keep individual variability to a minimum, muscle testing should always be performed by the same examiner. If possible, testing should not be performed by the patient's therapist, because he or she is usually unable to make an unbiased evaluation.
- Passive range of motion must be tested prior to determining the strength grade. The therapist must take any range-of-motion restrictions into account and note them in the evaluation. Restrictions may be related to the joints (ligament, capsule), bones, muscles, or nerves. Joint status, as measured by the neutral zero method, must be included if the normal range of motion cannot be achieved for these reasons.
- The examiner must adjust the level of resistance to the patient's constitution, age, and sex, and to the functions being tested. For instance, the examiner should apply more resistance with an active athlete than with an out-of-shape older adult. The examiner should apply less force when testing distal thumb extension than when examining elbow flexion. In case of doubt, the examiner can use the patient's healthy side to determine the individual's maximum strength.
- The examiner must record the final muscle testing results on a scoring sheet.
- This system cannot be used for testing patients with spasticity.

Evaluating Muscle Strength

0 = No visible or palpable contraction of a muscle involved in the movement.

1 = Visible or palpable contraction of a muscle that participates in the movement or the partially performed movement being tested, when the force of gravity is minimized.

The examiner can test the muscle's tension by palpating its origin, insertion, or muscle belly.

In some cases, it is easier to detect contraction when a muscle's insertion and origin are close together.

Images with palpation points for muscle testing are presented throughout this book.

If the examiner has doubts about the innervation of a muscle involved in a movement, the muscle must be tested while it is performing its primary action.

Some muscles cannot be palpated, owing to their anatomical position. These muscles are listed in the sections below.

2 = The muscle can complete the full range of motion when the force of gravity is minimized.

To reduce movement-related friction as much as possible, the examiner should place a cloth between the body part being tested and the testing surface.

3 = The muscle can complete the full range of motion against the resistance of gravity.

4 = The muscle can complete the full range of motion against the resistance of gravity and against moderate resistance (adjusted to the patient and movement being evaluated).

5 = The muscle can complete the full range of motion against the resistance of gravity and against maximum resistance (adjusted to the patient and to the movement being tested) (Janda 2009, Montgomery and Hislop 2007).

6 = The muscle can complete the full range of motion against the resistance of gravity and against maximum resistance and can perform the movement at least 10 times. By having the patient perform 10 repetitions, the examiner can make a fairly reliable statement about the muscle's strength endurance. "Strength endurance refers to the

neuromuscular system's ability to produce the greatest possible number of impulses in a defined time period (no longer than 2 minutes with maximal exertion) against higher loads (more than 30% of maximum strength) and, in so doing, keep the magnitude of the impulses as low as possible during the loading period" (Schmidt-bleicher 1989).

In their everyday lives, patients generally need strength endurance rather than maximum strength. For this reason, it makes sense to add a grade to the existing grading scale for muscle testing, in order to take this muscle activity into consideration.

If the muscle tested falls within this strength grade, it is difficult to manually determine the transition to normal strength (the individual's maximum strength). This can be measured in more detail with isokinetic strength testing.

Manual resistance must be used for grades 3, 4, 5, and 6, if the examiner cannot use gravity for testing.

If the strength level is between two grades, the examiner should record the lower grade.

Documenting Muscle Function

A scoring sheet is required for clear and informative documentation (see pp. 6–16). Apart from the patient's personal data, the sheet must include the following information:

- Which muscles are innervated and therefore perform the movement? Place a cross on the line corresponding to the muscle in question.
- At what strength level is a movement performed? Do the muscles exhibit a certain level of endurance? Enter the grade on a scale of 0 to 6 on the movement line.
- The examiner should note which spinal cord segment innervates a muscle and which peripheral nerve is responsible for innervation.
- The examiner must also write down the test dates and the name of the examiner.

Name of patient: _____

Date of birth: _____

Diagnosis: _____

Name of examiner: _____

	Left side		Right side	
	Date:		Date:	

Cervical spine extension

Cervical portion of autochthonous back muscles, C1–C8, dorsal branches of spinal nerves

Thoracic spine extension

Thoracic portion of autochthonous back muscles, T1–T12, dorsal branches of spinal nerves

Lumbar spine extension

Lumbar portion of autochthonous back muscles, L1–L5, dorsal branches of spinal nerves

Cervical spine flexion

Sternocleidomastoid muscle, accessory nerve, cervical plexus (C1–C2)

Rectus capitis anterior muscle, cervical plexus (C1–C4)

Longus capitis muscle, cervical plexus (C1–C4)

Longus colli muscle, brachial plexus, cervical plexus (C2–C8)

Trunk flexion

Rectus abdominis muscle, T5–T12, intercostal nerves

External and internal abdominal oblique muscles, T5–T12, intercostal nerves

Rotation of the trunk to the right

External abdominal oblique muscle, T5–T12, intercostal nerves

Internal abdominal oblique muscle, T10–T12, intercostal nerves and L1

Rotation of the trunk to the left									
External abdominal oblique muscle, T5–T12, intercostal nerves									
Internal abdominal oblique muscle, T10–T12, intercostal nerves and L1									
Lateral bending of the trunk									
Erector spinae muscles, C1–S4, dorsal branches of spinal nerves									
External abdominal oblique muscle, T5–T12, intercostal nerves									
Internal abdominal oblique muscle, T10–T12, intercostal nerves and L1									
Rectus abdominis muscle, T5–T12, intercostal nerves									
Latissimus dorsi muscle, C6–C8, thoracodorsal nerve									
Quadratus lumborum muscle, T12, intercostal nerve, L1–L3, lumbar plexus									

Name of patient: _____

Date of birth: _____

Diagnosis: _____

Name of examiner: _____

	Right side						Muscle	Left side					
Date:								Date:					
							Shoulder blade, cranially						
							Trapezius muscle, descending part, accessory nerve, trapezius branch (C2–C4)						
							Levator scapulae muscle, C4–C5, dorsal scapular nerve						
							Shoulder blade, caudally						
							Trapezius muscle, ascending part, accessory nerve, trapezius branch (C2–C4)						
							Serratus anterior muscle, C5–C7, long thoracic nerve						
							Shoulder blade, dorsally and medially						
							Trapezius muscle, accessory nerve, trapezius branch (C2–C4)						
							Rhomboid muscles, C4–C5, dorsal scapular nerve						
							Latissimus dorsi muscle, C6–C8, thoracodorsal nerve						
							Shoulder blade, ventrally and laterally						
							Serratus anterior muscle, C5–C7, long thoracic nerve						
							Pectoralis major and minor muscles, C5–T1, pectoral nerves						
							Shoulder joint, elevation						
							Deltoid muscle, clavicular part, C4–C6, axillary nerve						
							Biceps brachii muscle, C5–C6, musculocutaneous nerve						

Shoulder joint, extension

Teres major muscle, C6–C7, thoracodorsal nerve						
Latissimus dorsi muscle, C6–C8, thoracodorsal nerve						
Triceps brachii, long head, C6–C8, radial nerve						
Deltoid muscle, spinal part, C4–C6, axillary nerve						

Shoulder joint abduction

Deltoid muscle, C4–C6, axillary nerve						
Supraspinatus muscle, C4–C6, suprascapular nerve						

Shoulder joint adduction

Pectoralis major muscle, C5–T1, pectoral nerves						
Triceps brachii, long head, C6–C8, radial nerve						
Teres major muscle, C6–C7, thoracodorsal nerve						
Latissimus dorsi muscle, C6–C8, thoracodorsal nerve						

Shoulder joint, external rotation

Infraspinatus muscle, C4–C6, suprascapular nerve						
Teres minor muscle, C5–C6, axillary nerve						

Shoulder joint, internal rotation

Subscapularis muscle, C5–C8, subscapular nerve						
Teres major muscle, C6–C7, thoracodorsal nerve						

Elbow joint, flexion																
Biceps brachii muscle, C5–C6, musculocutaneous nerve																
Brachialis muscle, C5–C6, musculocutaneous nerve																
Brachioradialis muscle, C5–C6, radial nerve																
Elbow joint, extension																
Triceps brachii muscle, C6–C8, radial nerve																
Elbow joint, supination																
Supinator muscle, C5–C6, radial nerve																
Biceps brachii muscle, C5–C6, musculocutaneous nerve																
Elbow joint, pronation																
Pronator quadratus muscle, C8–T1, median nerve																
Pronator teres muscle, C6–C7, median nerve																
Wrist, extension																
Extensor digitorum communis muscle, C6–C8, radial nerve																
Extensor carpi radialis longus muscle, C5–C7, radial nerve																
Extensor indicis muscle, C6–C8, radial nerve																
Extensor carpi radialis brevis muscle, C5–C7, radial nerve																

Wrist, flexion

Flexor digitorum superficialis muscle, C7–T1, median nerve

Flexor digitorum profundus muscle, C7–T1, median nerve, ulnar nerve

Flexor carpi ulnaris muscle, C7–C8, ulnar nerve

Flexor pollicis longus, C7–C8, median nerve

Flexor carpi radialis muscle, C6–C7, median nerve

Wrist joint, ulnar abduction

Extensor carpi ulnaris muscle, C7–C8, radial nerve

Flexor carpi ulnaris muscle, C7–C8, ulnar nerve

Finger flexion/metacarpophalangeal (MCP)

Dorsal and palmar interossei muscles, C8–T1, ulnar nerve

Lumbrical muscles, C8–T1, median nerve, ulnar nerve

Flexor digitorum superficialis muscle, C7–T1, median nerve

Flexor digitorum profundus muscle, C7–T1, median nerve, ulnar nerve

Finger flexion/proximal interphalangeal joint (PIP)

Flexor digitorum superficialis muscle, C7–T1, median nerve

Flexor digitorum profundus muscle, C7–T1, median nerve, ulnar nerve

Finger flexion/distal interphalangeal joint (DIP)

Flexor digitorum profundus muscle, C7–T1, median nerve, ulnar nerve

Finger extension/MCP									
Extensor digitorum communis muscle, C6–C8, radial nerve									
Extensor indicis muscle, C6–C8, radial nerve									
Extensor digiti minimi muscle, C6–C8, radial nerve									
Finger extension/PIP and DIP									
Extensor digitorum communis muscle, C6–C8, radial nerve									
Extensor indicis muscle, C6–C8, radial nerve									
Extensor digiti minimi muscle, C6–C8, radial nerve									
Dorsal and palmar interossei muscles, C8–T1, ulnar nerve									
Finger spreading									
Dorsal interossei muscles, C8–T1, ulnar nerve									
Abductor digiti minimi muscle, C8–T1, ulnar nerve									
Finger closing									
Palmar interossei muscles, C8–T1, ulnar nerve									
Thumb flexion, carpometacarpal joint									
Flexor pollicis longus muscle, C7–C8, median nerve									
Flexor pollicis brevis muscle, C8–T1, median nerve, ulnar nerve									
Abductor pollicis brevis muscle, C8–T1, median nerve									
Opponens pollicis muscle, C6–C7, median nerve									

Thumb flexion, metacarpophalangeal joint								
Flexor pollicis longus muscle, *C7–C8*, median nerve								
Flexor pollicis brevis muscle, *C8–T1*, median nerve, ulnar nerve								
Thumb flexion, interphalangeal joint								
Flexor pollicis longus muscle, *C7–C8*, median nerve								
Thumb extension, carpometacarpal joint								
Extensor pollicis longus muscle, *C7–C8*, radial nerve								
Extensor pollicis brevis muscle, *C7–T1*, radial nerve								
Abductor pollicis longus muscle, *C7–C8*, radial nerve								
Thumb extension, metacarpophalangeal joint								
Extensor pollicis longus muscle, *C7–C8*, radial nerve								
Extensor pollicis brevis muscle, *C7–T1*, radial nerve								
Thumb extension, interphalangeal joint								
Extensor pollicis longus muscle, *C7–C8*, radial nerve								
Thumb adduction, carpometacarpal joint								
Adductor pollicis muscle, *C8–T1*, ulnar nerve								
Flexor pollicis brevis muscle, *C8–T1*, ulnar nerve								
Thumb abduction, carpometacarpal joint								
Abductor pollicis longus muscle, *C7–C8*, radial nerve								
Abductor pollicis brevis muscle, *C8–T1*, median nerve								

Name of patient: _____

Date of birth: _____

Diagnosis: _____

Name of examiner: _____

Right side — Date: ___

Left side — Date: ___

Hip joint flexion

Iliopsoas muscle, L1–L4, lumbar plexus, femoral nerve

Rectus femoris muscle, L2–L4, femoral nerve

Sartorius muscle, L1–L3, femoral nerve

Hip joint extension

Gluteus maximus muscle, L5–S2, inferior gluteal nerve

Semimembranosus and semitendinosus muscles, L5–S2, tibial nerve

Gluteus medius and minimus muscles, L4–S1, superior gluteal nerve

Adductor magnus muscle, L3–L5, obturator nerve, tibial nerve

Biceps femoris muscle, long head, L5–S2, tibial nerve

Hip joint adduction

Adductor muscles, L2–L5, obturator nerve, tibial nerve

Gluteus maximus muscle, L5–S2, inferior gluteal nerve

Semimembranosus and semitendinosus muscles, L5–S2, tibial nerve

| **Hip joint abduction** |
| Gluteus medius and minimus muscles, L4–S1, superior gluteal nerve |
| Tensor of fascia lata muscle, L4–L5, superior gluteal nerve |
| Gluteus maximus muscle, L5–S2, inferior gluteal nerve |
| **Hip joint, external rotation** |
| Gluteus maximus muscle, L5–S2, inferior gluteal nerve |
| Gluteus medius and minimus muscles, dorsal portion, L4–S1, superior gluteal nerve |
| Short external rotators, L1–S2, obturator nerve, inferior gluteal nerve, sacral plexus |
| **Hip joint, internal rotation** |
| Gluteus medius and minimus muscles, L4–S1, superior gluteal nerve |
| Tensor of fascia lata muscle, L4–L5, superior gluteal nerve |
| **Knee joint extension** |
| Quadriceps femoris muscle, L2–L4, femoral nerve |
| **Knee joint flexion** |
| Semimembranosus and semitendinosus muscles, L5–S2, tibial nerve |
| Biceps femoris muscle, L5–S2, tibial nerve, and peroneal nerve |
| **Foot, plantar flexion** |
| Triceps surae muscle, S1–S2, tibial nerve |

Foot, dorsal extension															
Tibialis anterior muscle, L4–L5, deep peroneal nerve															
Extensor digitorum longus muscle, L5–S1, deep peroneal nerve															
Extensor hallucis longus muscle, L4–S1, deep peroneal nerve															
Foot pronation															
Peroneus longus and brevis muscles, L5–S1, superficial peroneal nerve															
Extensor digitorum longus muscle, L5–S1, deep peroneal nerve															
Foot supination															
Triceps surae muscle, S1–S2, tibial nerve															
Tibialis posterior muscle, L4–L5, tibial nerve															
Tibialis anterior muscle, L4–L5, deep peroneal nerve															
Toe flexion															
Flexor digitorum longus muscle, S1–S3, tibial nerve															
Flexor digitorum brevis muscle, L5–S1, medial plantar nerve															
Big toe flexion															
Flexor hallucis longus and brevis muscles, L5–S3, tibial nerve, medial plantar nerve															
Toe extension															
Extensor digitorum longus and brevis muscles, L5–S2, deep peroneal nerve															
Big toe extension															
Extensor hallucis longus and brevis muscles, L4–S2, deep peroneal nerve															

Diagnosis at the Neurological Level

When examining patients with neurological deficits, the damaged region must be precisely identified. A distinction is made between damage to the central nervous system and to the peripheral nervous system. For both types of damage, the injury site should be determined as accurately as possible.

Central efferent pathways are used to describe the pyramidal system (**Fig. 1**), which originates in the primary motor cortex of the brain. This system encompasses the lateral corticospinal tract, which supplies the hand and foot muscles and distal arm and leg muscles; the anterior corticospinal tract, which supplies the neck and trunk muscles and proximal arm and leg muscles; and the corticonuclear tract, which supplies the motor nuclei of the cranial nerves, except for those of the eye mus-

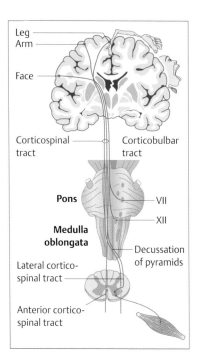

Fig. 1 Motor system: pyramidal tract and somatotropic representation of the skeletal musculature in the primary motor cortex (motor homunculus).

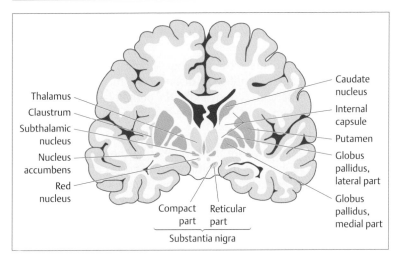

Thalamus

Claustrum

Subthalamic
nucleus

Nucleus
accumbens

Red
nucleus

Compact   Reticular
part   part

Substantia nigra

Caudate
nucleus

Internal
capsule

Putamen

Globus
pallidus,
lateral part

Globus
pallidus,
medial part

Fig. 2   The basal ganglia comprise subcortical nuclei in the telencephalon. They play a role in planning and performing movements.

cles. The three tracts have a common course through the internal capsule into the cerebral penduncles, where the corticonuclear tract branches off. The corticospinal tracts pass through the medulla oblongata. At the transition to the spinal cord, the lateral corticospinal tract crosses to the opposite side, while the anterior corticospinal tract does not switch to the other side until it reaches the level of the respective target segment. The lateral pyramidal tract is primarily responsible for the target motor function of the distal extremities, while the anterior pyramidal tract is responsible for postural reflexes and trunk movements, and for stabilizing body posture during arm and leg movements. Other systems, particularly the subcortical motor system, also impinge on these movement sequences controlled by the pyramidal system. The subcortical motor system comprises the striatum (caudate nucleus, putamen), the subthalamic nucleus, and the substantia nigra (**Fig. 2**). The subcortical centers are connected with each other in different ways and are also connected to the cerebral cortex, in order to inhibit or promote motor function (**Fig. 3**) (Rohen 2001). The peripheral motor system begins with the anterior horn motor neuron and its distal processes. Central and peripheral nervous system disorders can be manifested as a change in muscle tone and monosynaptic reflexes. Damage to the spinal cord or the peripheral nervous system is usually also manifested as sensory disorders (see **Figs. 5–8**).

Increased muscle tone is always a sign of a central nervous system disorder, except in the early stages of a stroke or quadriplegia. In these conditions, muscle tone is reduced but, later on, muscle tone increases as well.

Peripheral lesions are always manifested by reduced muscle tone, flaccid paralysis, and muscle atrophy (Duus 2012). In both cases, monosynaptic reflexes change in the same manner as muscle tone, that is, reflexes increase with increased muscle tone and decrease with reduced muscle tone. For disorders of the central nervous system, such as quadriplegia, as well as disorders of the peripheral nervous system, such as cervical or lumbar disk herniation, the lesion level must be determined. For peripheral disorders, a further distinction must be made between the nerve root and the peripheral nerve.

By testing
- *muscle strength* and the *key muscles*
- *sensitivity to pain* and *cutaneous sensitivity*
- as well as *monosynaptic reflexes,*
the damaged region can be located easily and accurately.

■ Muscle Strength and Key Muscles

Fig. 3 presents a schematic diagram of *motor innervation.* It clearly shows the topographic relationship of the spinal cord segments to the vertebral segments. In the upper part of the spinal column, the spinal cord segment and vertebrae are located at approximately the same level; in the lower part of the spinal column, this is not the case. For example, the fifth lumbar segment is located between the T11 and T12 vertebrae. This is the result of the vertebral column growing more rapidly and becoming longer than the spinal cord during development.

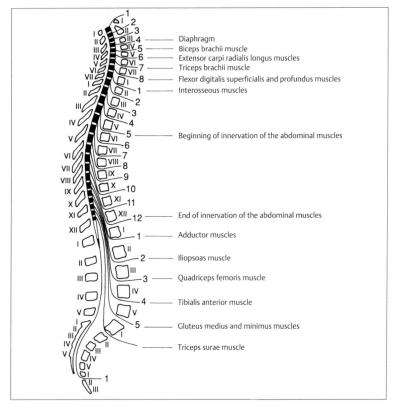

Fig. 3   Schematic diagram of segmental innervation with key muscles.

The muscles depicted in **Fig. 4 a, b** are referred to as *key muscles.* For the most part, their innervation can be assigned to a specific spinal cord segment. When these muscles are tested, they can be assigned to a segmental level. In a patient with spinal cord injury, if the triceps brachii is still innervated but the key muscles below the C7 level are no longer active, this is referred to as complete spinal cord injury below C7. When a patient with a lumbar disk herniation has a weak tibialis anterior muscle, the damage always affects the L4 nerve roots.

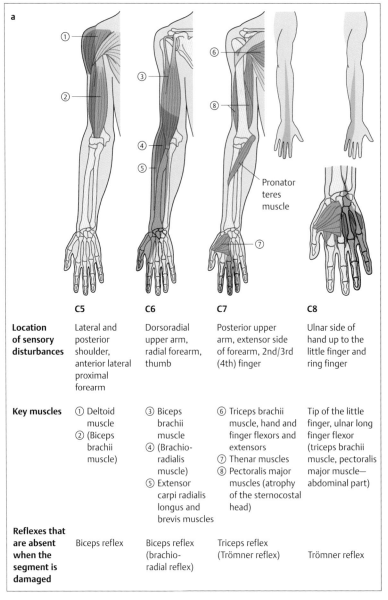

	C5	C6	C7	C8
Location of sensory disturbances	Lateral and posterior shoulder, anterior lateral proximal forearm	Dorsoradial upper arm, radial forearm, thumb	Posterior upper arm, extensor side of forearm, 2nd/3rd (4th) finger	Ulnar side of hand up to the little finger and ring finger
Key muscles	① Deltoid muscle ② (Biceps brachii muscle)	③ Biceps brachii muscle ④ (Brachioradialis muscle) ⑤ Extensor carpi radialis longus and brevis muscles	⑥ Triceps brachii muscle, hand and finger flexors and extensors ⑦ Thenar muscles ⑧ Pectoralis major muscles (atrophy of the sternocostal head)	Tip of the little finger, ulnar long finger flexor (triceps brachii muscle, pectoralis major muscle—abdominal part)
Reflexes that are absent when the segment is damaged	Biceps reflex	Biceps reflex (brachioradial reflex)	Triceps reflex (Trömner reflex)	Trömner reflex

Fig. 4 a Schematic diagram of segmental innervation of the upper extremity, with key muscles, reflexes, and sensations.

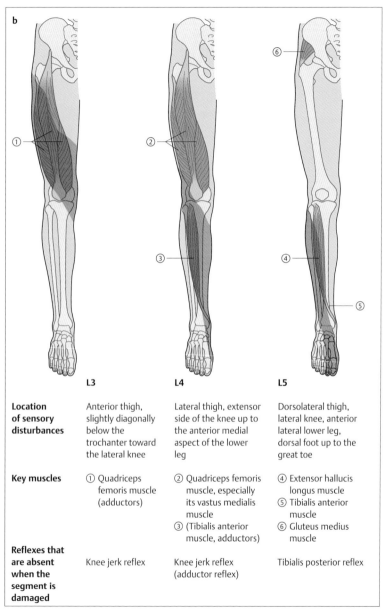

	L3	**L4**	**L5**
Location of sensory disturbances	Anterior thigh, slightly diagonally below the trochanter toward the lateral knee	Lateral thigh, extensor side of the knee up to the anterior medial aspect of the lower leg	Dorsolateral thigh, lateral knee, anterior lateral lower leg, dorsal foot up to the great toe
Key muscles	① Quadriceps femoris muscle (adductors)	② Quadriceps femoris muscle, especially its vastus medialis muscle ③ (Tibialis anterior muscle, adductors)	④ Extensor hallucis longus muscle ⑤ Tibialis anterior muscle ⑥ Gluteus medius muscle
Reflexes that are absent when the segment is damaged	Knee jerk reflex	Knee jerk reflex (adductor reflex)	Tibialis posterior reflex

Fig. 4 b   Schematic diagram of segmental innervation of the lower extremity, with key muscles, reflexes, and sensations.

■ Sensitivity to Pain and Cutaneous Sensitivity

The *sensory innervation scheme* is also used to more precisely locate the lesion. **Figs. 5–8** depict segmental and peripheral sensory innervation. Sensitivity to touch and pain is the easiest to test. In patients with a central nervous system disorder where the cutaneous sensitivity pathways are also affected, the deficits (anesthesia and analgesia) are widespread below the lesion. In patients with hemiparesis, the entire contralateral half of the body can be affected, because the sensory tracts generally switch to the opposite side at the segmental level (**Fig. 9**). Patients with complete spinal cord injury are completely insensitive to touch and pain below the lesion. Disk herniation at the L5 nerve root is characterized by paresthesia or anesthesia in the L5 dermatome. In this case, testing for pain sensation, which is also reduced or eliminated in the corresponding dermatome, is more reliable than testing for tactile sensation (**Fig. 10**). If the lesion is more peripheral, which is the case with a compressed nerve, hypoesthesia and hypoalgesia (or anesthesia and analgesia) will be present in the dermatome innervated by the nerve. In this case, testing for tactile sensation is more accurate, since the individual cutaneous nerves are more sharply delineated than the dermatomes, which can greatly overlap for cutaneous sensitivity (Duus 2012). The examiner tests tactile sensation by lightly touching the skin with the fingertips, or with the brush from the reflex hammer. A pin prick is used to test pain sensation.

On the trunk, the examiner pricks the skin from top to bottom and on the extremities, in a circular pattern, to ensure that the dermatomes are compared.

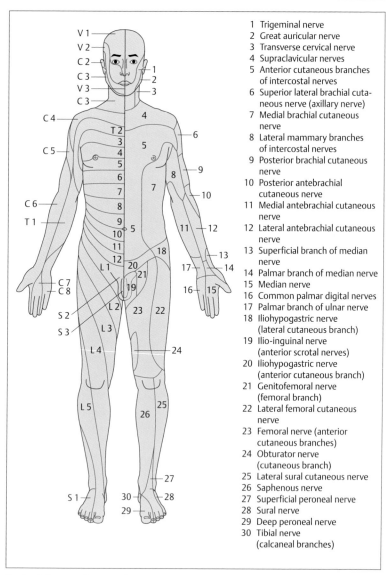

1 Trigeminal nerve
2 Great auricular nerve
3 Transverse cervical nerve
4 Supraclavicular nerves
5 Anterior cutaneous branches of intercostal nerves
6 Superior lateral brachial cutaneous nerve (axillary nerve)
7 Medial brachial cutaneous nerve
8 Lateral mammary branches of intercostal nerves
9 Posterior brachial cutaneous nerve
10 Posterior antebrachial cutaneous nerve
11 Medial antebrachial cutaneous nerve
12 Lateral antebrachial cutaneous nerve
13 Superficial branch of median nerve
14 Palmar branch of median nerve
15 Median nerve
16 Common palmar digital nerves
17 Palmar branch of ulnar nerve
18 Iliohypogastric nerve (lateral cutaneous branch)
19 Ilio-inguinal nerve (anterior scrotal nerves)
20 Iliohypogastric nerve (anterior cutaneous branch)
21 Genitofemoral nerve (femoral branch)
22 Lateral femoral cutaneous nerve
23 Femoral nerve (anterior cutaneous branches)
24 Obturator nerve (cutaneous branch)
25 Lateral sural cutaneous nerve
26 Saphenous nerve
27 Superficial peroneal nerve
28 Sural nerve
29 Deep peroneal nerve
30 Tibial nerve (calcaneal branches)

Fig. 5 Schematic diagram of sensory innervation, anterior view: right side, segmental innervation; left side, peripheral innervation.

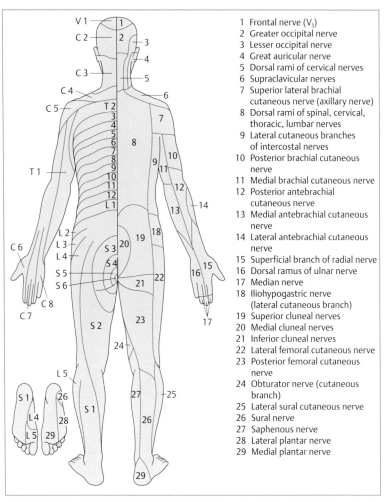

1 Frontal nerve (V₁)
2 Greater occipital nerve
3 Lesser occipital nerve
4 Great auricular nerve
5 Dorsal rami of cervical nerves
6 Supraclavicular nerves
7 Superior lateral brachial cutaneous nerve (axillary nerve)
8 Dorsal rami of spinal, cervical, thoracic, lumbar nerves
9 Lateral cutaneous branches of intercostal nerves
10 Posterior brachial cutaneous nerve
11 Medial brachial cutaneous nerve
12 Posterior antebrachial cutaneous nerve
13 Medial antebrachial cutaneous nerve
14 Lateral antebrachial cutaneous nerve
15 Superficial branch of radial nerve
16 Dorsal ramus of ulnar nerve
17 Median nerve
18 Iliohypogastric nerve (lateral cutaneous branch)
19 Superior cluneal nerves
20 Medial cluneal nerves
21 Inferior cluneal nerves
22 Lateral femoral cutaneous nerve
23 Posterior femoral cutaneous nerve
24 Obturator nerve (cutaneous branch)
25 Lateral sural cutaneous nerve
26 Sural nerve
27 Saphenous nerve
28 Lateral plantar nerve
29 Medial plantar nerve

Fig. 6　Schematic diagram of sensory innervation, posterior view: right side, peripheral innervation; left side, segmental innervation.

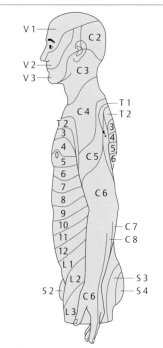

1 Ilio-inguinal nerve
2 Iliohypogastric nerve
3 Genitofemoral nerve (femoral branch)
4 Lateral femoral cutaneous nerve
5 Dorsal nerve of penis (pudendal nerve)
6 Trigeminal nerve/1
7 Trigeminal nerve/3
8 Lesser occipital nerve
9 Trigeminal nerve/2
10 Greater occipital nerve
11 Dorsal rami of cervical nerves
12 Great auricular nerve
13 Transverse cervical nerve
14 Anterior cutaneous branches of
    intercostal nerves
15 Supraclavicular nerves
16 Superior lateral brachial cutaneous
    nerve (axillary nerve)
17 Intercostobrachial nerves
    (intercostal nerves)

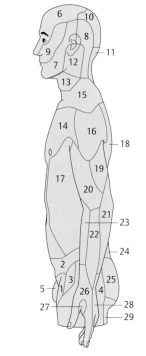

18 Dorsal rami of thoracic nerves
19 Posterior brachial cutaneous nerve
20 Lateral brachial cutaneous nerve
21 Posterior antebrachial cutaneous
    nerve (radial nerve)
22 Superior lateral antebrachial
    cutaneous nerve
23 Medial antebrachial cutaneous nerve
24 Lateral cutaneous branch of
    iliohypogastric nerve
25 Superior cluneal nerves
26 Superficial branch of radial nerve
27 Autonomic region of the superficial
    branch radial nerve
28 Dorsal ramus of ulnar nerve
29 Inferior cluneal nerve
30 Median common digital palmar
    nerve

Fig. 7 Lateral view, segmental innervation.　　**Fig. 8** Lateral view, peripheral innervation.

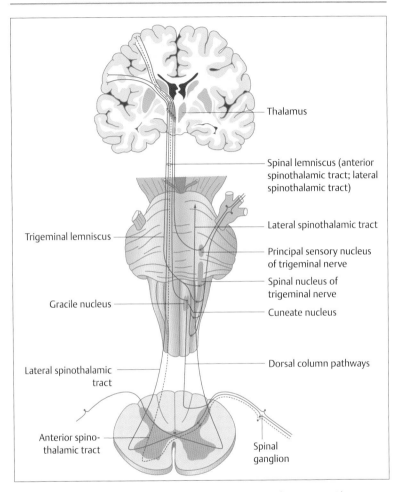

Fig. 9 Course of the sensory pathways, which can cross over to the opposite side at segmental level.

Thalamus

Spinal lemniscus (anterior spinothalamic tract; lateral spinothalamic tract)

Lateral spinothalamic tract

Principal sensory nucleus of trigeminal nerve

Spinal nucleus of trigeminal nerve

Cuneate nucleus

Dorsal column pathways

Spinal ganglion

Trigeminal lemniscus

Gracile nucleus

Lateral spinothalamic tract

Anterior spino-thalamic tract

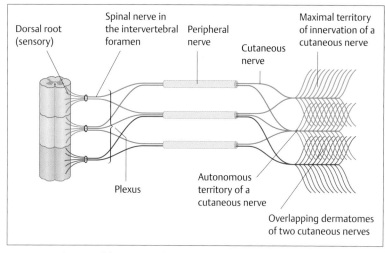

Fig. 10   Overlapping of dermatomes from adjacent posterior roots (cutaneous sensitivity).

■ Monosynaptic Reflexes

Reflex testing is another important criterion for evaluating cervical and lumbar disk herniation. If the disk protrudes or is prolapsed (peripheral damage), the monosynaptic reflexes for the corresponding level will be diminished or absent compared to the healthy side, depending on the severity of the disturbance. In the cervical spine, segments C5, C6, and C7 are tested, while in the lumbar spine, segments L3, L4, L5, and S1 are tested (**Figs. 11– 16**).

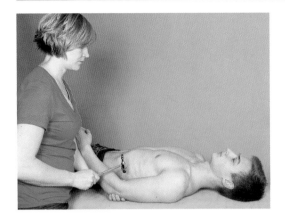

Fig. 11   Testing of the biceps reflex (neurological level C5). The patient lies supine. The examiner holds the patient's slightly flexed arm with the examiner's hand, so that he or she can place the thumb on the biceps tendon in the area of the elbow, and the forearm lies relaxed on the patient's body. The examiner strikes the thumb with the reflex hammer. Reflexes are normal if they show slight contraction in the area of the biceps brachii.

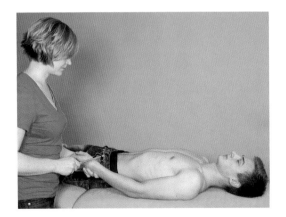

Fig. 12   Testing of the brachioradialis reflex (neurological level C6). The patient lies supine. The examiner holds the patient's arm with the elbow flexed. The examiner strikes the brachioradialis muscle tendon with the reflex hammer directly proximal to its insertion at the radial styloid process. The normal reflex response is slight contraction in the direction of elbow flexion.

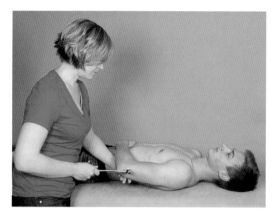

Fig. 13   Testing of the triceps reflex (neurological level C7). The patient lies supine. The examiner holds the patient's arm with the elbow flexed and strikes the triceps brachii tendon with the reflex hammer directly above the olecranon. If the reflex is normal, muscle contraction can be seen or felt.

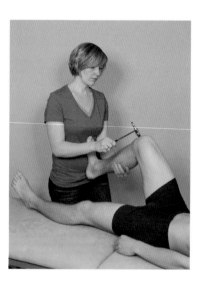

Fig. 14   Testing of the knee-jerk reflex (neurological level L3 and L4). The patient lies supine, with the leg to be tested pressed against the examiner's abdomen, with the hip and knee slightly flexed. The examiner supports the leg with one hand in the popliteal fossa. The examiner strikes the patellar tendon with the reflex hammer between the tibial tuberosity and the patella. This should cause a quadriceps contraction and a sudden leg extension.

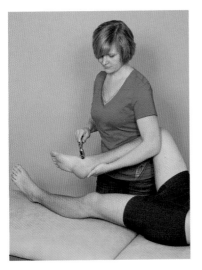

Fig. 15 Testing of the tibialis posterior reflex (neurological level L5). The patient lies supine. The examiner holds the patient's leg with the hip and knee flexed. The patient's foot is slightly pronated. The examiner strikes the tibialis posterior muscle tendon between the medial malleolus and its insertion at the navicular tuberosity. The normal reflex response is a slight contraction toward supination of the foot. It is difficult to elicit the tibialis posterior reflex.

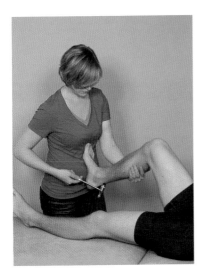

Fig. 16 Testing of the ankle-jerk reflex (neurological level S1). The patient lies supine, with the leg to be tested pressed against the examiner's abdomen, with the hip and knee slightly flexed. The patient's ankle is dorsiflexed. The examiner holds the patient's leg with one hand and with the other hand taps the Achilles tendon with the reflex hammer. Under normal circumstances, the foot should jerk in the direction of plantar flexion (Hoppenfeld 1980).

To perform reflex testing and evaluate the results, the examiner requires a certain amount of practice, as well as familiarity with the anatomical details. During reflex testing, the patient should be as relaxed as possible. For this reason, the supine position is the position of choice for most of the reflex tests.

However, it is not the reflex testing per se but rather the interpretation of the results that is challenging. For example, in addition to comparing the extremities on both sides, the upper extremity has to be compared to the lower extremity, since some patients have an overall tendency toward sluggish or hyperactive reflexes. Furthermore, numerous potential sources of error need to be minimized. The muscle being tested must be stretched slightly before it is tested. However, any change to the joint position will also affect the magnitude of the reflex. The examiner can place a thumb on thin tendons and then strike the thumb, in order to elicit the reflex. Here also, the thumb pressure must be consistent; otherwise the muscle spindle's stretch will be altered and will produce a different result. If the reflex is very difficult to elicit, the examiner can ask the patient to contract the muscle against resistance and then test it again.

Examples of Central Nervous System Disturbances

The following symptoms are signs of central spastic paralysis (Duus 2012):

- diminished strength, accompanied by disturbed fine motor function
- increased muscle tone
- increased reflex activity
- pathological reflexes, with diminished or absent monosynaptic reflexes and no degenerative muscle atrophy.

■ Complete Spinal Cord Injury below C6

Manual muscle testing. The deepest key muscles that can be tested are the extensor carpi radialis longus and the extensor carpi radialis brevis, both of which may have reduced strength. Initially, there is flaccid paralysis below the level of the lesion (spinal shock). In this phase, there is no muscle activity. Later, spastic paralysis develops, that is, uncontrolled increase in muscle activity.

Sensory testing. There is hypersensitivity in the dermatome at the level of the lesion and a complete absence of all sensory qualities below the level of the lesion.

Monosynaptic reflexes. The biceps reflex (C5) can be elicited normally, while the brachioradialis reflex (C6) may be somewhat diminished. The triceps reflex (C7) and all monosynaptic reflexes are absent in the flaccid phase and are excessive in the spastic phase.

■ Right Hemiplegia (Brain Damage to the Left Hemisphere)

Manual muscle testing. Muscle testing cannot be performed. In the initial phase, flaccid paralysis occurs that changes to spasticity at a later stage (increased uncontrolled muscle activity). Motor functions vary widely, depending on the damage.

Sensory testing. Tactile and pain sensations are more or less disturbed, depending on the degree of damage. In patients with this condition, it is important to test proprioception and body perception. A more detailed discussion of these specific tests is beyond the scope of this book.

Monosynaptic reflexes. In the flaccid phase, there is areflexia; in the later stages, there is hyperreflexia in the spastic muscle groups.

Examples of Peripheral Damage

The following symptoms are signs of peripheral flaccid paralysis (Duus 2012):

- reduced strength or complete loss of strength
- reduced muscle tone
- diminished or absent muscle reflexes
- muscle atrophy.

Herniated Disk L4–L5 (Root Compression L4)

Manual muscle testing. The strength of the quadriceps femoris and tibialis anterior muscles is reduced.

Sensory testing. In the L4 dermatome, sensation is reduced or absent. Testing for pain sensation produces considerably more reliable results than testing for tactile sensation (see p. 23).

Monosynaptic reflexes. The knee-jerk reflex is diminished.

Foraminal Stenosis C5–C6, e.g., due to Osteochondrosis (Root Compression of C6 Nerve Root)

Manual muscle testing. The strength of the biceps brachii and the brachioradialis muscles is significantly diminished.

Sensory testing. In the C6 dermatome, sensation is reduced or absent.

Monosynaptic reflexes. The biceps or brachioradialis reflex is affected.

■ Injury to the Radial Nerve in the Lower Third of the Humeral Shaft

Manual muscle testing. The triceps brachii muscle will have normal strength. The hand and finger extensors and the brachioradialis muscle present with flaccid paralysis (no muscle activity).

Sensory testing. There is a loss of cutaneous sensitivity in the area supplied by the posterior cutaneous nerve of the forearm and the thumb and dorsal hand.

Monosynaptic reflexes. While the triceps reflex can be elicited normally, the brachioradialis reflex is absent.

■ Poliomyelitis (Inflammation of the Anterior Horn, Peripheral Nervous System)

Manual muscle testing. Flaccid paralysis is present (no muscle activity in the area supplied by the inflamed spinal cord segments).

Sensory testing. Sensation is not disturbed because only the anterior horn motor neurons are affected by the inflammation.

Monosynaptic reflexes. Reflex activity is absent in the affected muscles.

■ Polyneuropathy

Deficits are usually bilateral and tend to occur in the distal parts of the extremities. They are characterized by motor, sensory, and autonomic deficits affecting several nerves. Often, there is stocking glove sensory loss, flaccid paralysis with considerable muscle atrophy, and trophic skin lesions. Since proprioception is also affected, patients report feeling unsteady when standing and walking.

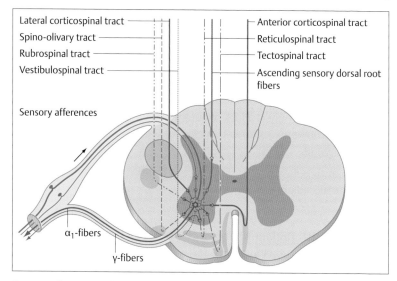

Lateral corticospinal tract
Spino-olivary tract
Rubrospinal tract
Vestibulospinal tract

Anterior corticospinal tract
Reticulospinal tract
Tectospinal tract
Ascending sensory dorsal root fibers

Sensory afferences

α_1-fibers

γ-fibers

Fig. 17   Influences on alpha and gamma motor neurons.

Muscle Synergy

Muscle synergy is defined as the proper coordination of different muscles when holding a position or during movements. It greatly influences the joint position and the loading or overloading of passive and active structures of the musculoskeletal system. Without teamwork between different muscles, the targeted movements cannot be performed.

If the C5 segment is in a lordotic position of the cervical spine, for example, owing to weak anterior cervical muscles, the disk in this segment will be subjected to shear forces more than pressure. In addition, the facet joints are also subjected to greater loads in this position. If this abnormal posture persists, the neck muscles will be constantly pressed together and will respond by shortening, which is the ultimate outcome of overloading (**Fig. 18**).

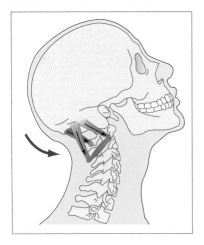

Fig. 18 Function of the short neck muscles: extension.

When performing a movement, a distinction is made between *agonists* and *antagonists*, as well as between *mover* and *stabilizer* muscles.

To better understand our daily movements, they can be broken down into simple, single-axis movements. Performing the desired action requires well-oiled muscle interactions. Very few muscles are positioned so that they can have a single-axis effect; that is, during flexion or extension of the hip, external or internal rotation and abduction or adduction are always present. Therefore, to perform pure flexion in a sagittal plane, muscles must rotate to correct this movement and must counteract and control the movement through abduction or adduction. In line with this, the external rotation components of the iliopsoas muscle counteract other muscles to maintain the movement in the desired plane. These muscles are referred to as *mover muscles*.

Stabilizer muscles are always needed when forces on an extremity need to be transferred to the trunk. Since nearly all muscles that flex the hip joint have their origin at the pelvic ring (except the psoas major and minor muscles), the pelvis must be stabilized to the trunk during hip joint flexion. This is primarily accomplished by the abdominal muscles. Without this stabilization, flexion could not be performed at full strength and the pelvis would be pulled into a tilted position with increased lumbar lordosis.

If the shoulder joint needs to be abducted, the full force of the deltoid and supraspinatus muscles will have only a minimal impact if the scapula is not sufficiently stabilized on the trunk by the scapula fixators (trapezius, serratus anterior, and rhomboid muscles) and the trunk muscles will then transfer the force to the pelvic girdle.

These elements must be kept in mind during muscle testing, especially for movements of the hip and shoulder joints. On the one hand, if the patient cannot perform a movement in one of these large joints at full strength, the examiner must determine whether the shoulder girdle or the pelvic girdle is being properly stablized. If this stability is absent, the examiner must manually apply it, in order to evaluate the joint movement somewhat objectively.

Disturbance of this muscle synergy is referred to as *muscular imbalance.* It can be caused by muscle weakness and/or muscle shortening. As described above, the consequences are overloading of passive and active structures of the musculoskeletal system, which can be manifested as degeneration or tendinopathy.

Grading for Manual Muscle Testing

Examining a patient encompasses several criteria, beginning with the patient's history, survey of the posture at rest, evaluation during active movement, gait analysis, and muscle testing, to name just a few. While each of these items yields certain information, the results are not informative or conclusive until all of this information is pulled together. Muscle testing is an especially important aspect for decoding individual pieces of information, in order to obtain a functionally complete picture of the patient.

If the patient reports weakness when climbing stairs, muscle testing can be used to establish whether this is caused by the calf muscles, the quadriceps, or the hip extensors. If the examiner observes genu recurvatum, muscle testing can be used to determine whether this condition is the result of weakness in the knee extensors or flexors. If the patient limps, the test can detect whether the limp is caused by muscular weakness or is due to pain.

When a patient makes compensatory movements of the shoulder girdle and has an incomplete range of motion (e.g., during arm flexion), a distinction must be made between weakness in the shoulder joint and in the shoulder girdle muscles. If both muscle groups have normal strength, the reason for this must be found elsewhere, for example, limited mobility in the shoulder joint due to capsular restriction or shortened muscles.

An efficiently conducted treatment (i.e., initiating treatment at the proper time) is in the best interests of both the patient and therapist. Muscle testing helps to detect and precisely evaluate any existing weaknesses. Deviations from normal movement can be explained and abnormal posture can be analyzed and the reasons identified. By repeating muscle testing at regular intervals, treatment success can be monitored.

2
Quick Tests for Evaluating Overall Muscle Function

When taking a patient's history, information is often elicited that indicates muscle weakness. In such cases, quick tests can be helpful for obtaining a broader overview of muscle function.

As the adjective "overall" indicates, the individual results of these general tests are not significant enough to be used as a basis for targeted treatment. However, they are useful in practice and can serve as a foundation for specific muscle testing.

All of the tests evaluate muscle strength, along with coordination and the neuromuscular system.

When the examiner performs only a quick test, he or she cannot necessarily assume, based on the test result, that the patient has diminished strength.

If the examiner observes weaknesses when the patient performs a test, the patient's coordination must be evaluated and specific muscle tests performed, in order to draw an accurate conclusion.

Matthiass Postural Competence Test for Children between 6 and 16 Years of Age

This test assesses the capacity of the trunk muscles, shoulder girdle muscles, and muscles that attach the scapula to the thorax (Matthiass 1979).

Procedure. The examination is performed with the patient standing. The patient is asked to raise the arms in front up to 90° and to hold this position for 30 seconds (**Fig. 19 a, b**).

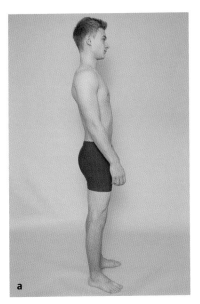
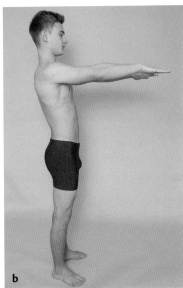

Fig. 19

Assessment. If the patient is able to maintain this position without changing it for the specified amount of time, he or she is considered to have "healthy posture."

If the patient changes position before the end of the test, by lowering the arms or bending the upper body backward (increasing lumbar lordosis), or not keeping the shoulder girdle retracted, the patient has first-degree postural weakness (**Fig. 20 a, b**).

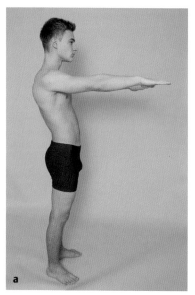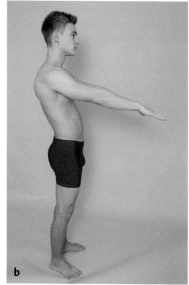

Fig. 20

If the patient is unable to fully reach the test position, he or she has second-degree postural weakness (**Fig. 21**) (Buckup 2008).

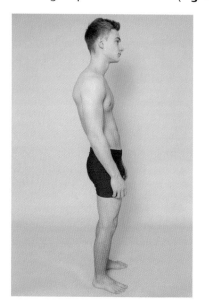

Fig. 21

Toe and Heel Walking Test

This test is performed to assess the general muscle strength of the foot dorsiflexors (heel walking) or of the calf muscles (toe walking) in patients such as those with a nerve root disorder in the lower lumbar spine.

Procedure. The patient is asked to walk around the room, first on the heels, then on the toes, shifting full weight from one leg to the other leg (**Fig. 22 a, b**).

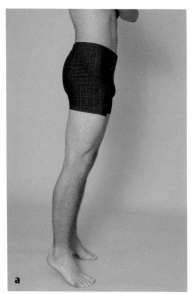
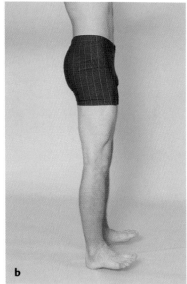

Fig. 22

Assessment. Difficulty standing on the heels without the forefoot dropping may suggest a lesion of the L4–L5 nerve root. Difficulty walking on the toes suggests a lesion of the S1 nerve root (Buckup 2008).

Standing on One Leg

This test provides information about the strength of the hip abductors.

Procedure. The patient stands on one leg without using the arms to stay upright. The patient must hold the pelvis in the horizontal plane without significantly shifting the center of gravity over the hip joint of the supporting leg (**Fig. 23 a**).

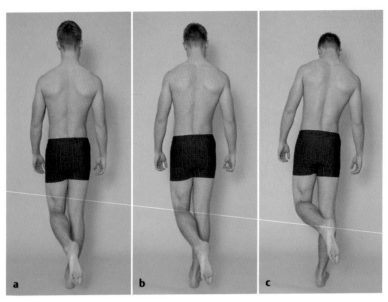

Fig. 23

Assessment. If the patient's muscles are weak, the pelvis on the side of the non-standing leg will drop, or the center of gravity will significantly shift over to the hip joint of the standing leg, so as to minimize the work being done by the abductors to hold the position (**Fig. 23 b, c**) (Buckup 2008).

Squat

The strength of the hip and knee extensors can be assessed by having the patient perform a squat.

Procedure. If possible, the patient should squat down and stand back up without holding on to anything (**Fig. 24 a, b**).

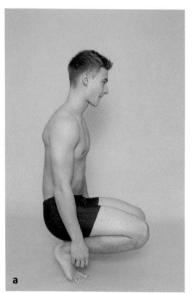 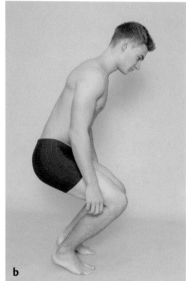

Fig. 24

Assessment. If there is a muscular weakness, the patient will attempt to support himself or herself by placing the hands on the thighs.

Push-up

The overall strength of the shoulder girdle, elbow extensors, and trunk muscles can be assessed by having the patient perform a push-up. Of course, the patient also needs to have sufficient strength in the pelvis and hips, as well as in the lower extremities (**Fig. 25 a**) to perform this movement.

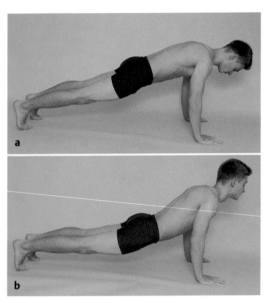

Fig. 25

Procedure. The patient places the hands shoulder distance apart, with the fingers pointing forward. The body and legs form a straight line and the balls of the feet are on the ground. From this position, the patient bends the arms until the upper arms are horizontal and then extends the arms again.

Assessment. Various signs of muscular weakness can be observed: insufficient flexion and extension of the arms (weak triceps brachii muscle or fixators of the scapula), sagging back (weak trunk muscles), change in the pelvis position (weak pelvis and hip muscles), or instability of the lower extremities (weak femoral quadriceps muscle, toe flexors, etc.) (**Fig. 25 b**).

Small children are sometimes unwilling to perform a push-up. In this case, the therapist can "wheelbarrow walk" the child instead. Younger patients seem to like this version of the test much better.

Step Test

The strength of the knee extensors and the hip abductors can be assessed by asking the patient to step up on a platform.

Procedure. The patient steps up onto a platform without holding onto anything (**Fig. 26**).

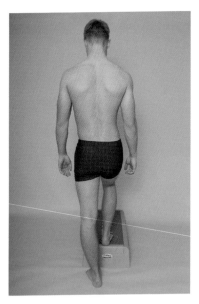

Fig. 26

Assessment. If the knee extensors are weak, the patient will support himself or herself by placing the hands on the thighs.

If the hip abductors are weak, the patient will not be able to hold the body centered and will shift his or her body weight over the test side.

Side Plank

The side plank is used to assess the strength of the lateral trunk muscles and hip abductors.

Procedure. The patient lies on one side and props himself or herself up on the forearm, pressing the body up sideways. The patient's trunk remains in a straight line (**Fig. 27 a**).

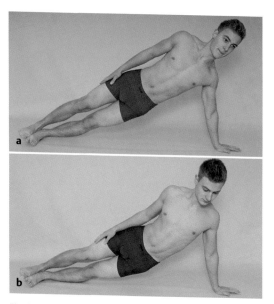

Fig. 27

Assessment. If the patient is unable to push up from the table, or if the pelvis drops, the trunk muscles are weak (**Fig. 27 b**).

3
Head and Face

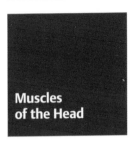

**Muscles
of the Head**

The muscles of the head can be divided into three main groups:

- muscles of mastication
- muscles of facial expression
- muscles of the eye.

The patient is supine while these muscles are palpated, with the examiner sitting at the head end of the table.

Muscles of Mastication

The muscles of mastication open and close the temporomandibular joint. Since they operate synergistically, they cannot be evaluated separately. All of the muscles are innervated by the mandibular nerve, which arises from the third branch of the trigeminal nerve (fifth cranial nerve) (**Figs. 28a, b** and **29a**).

■ Masseter Muscle and Temporal Muscle (Fig. 28a, b)

Muscle	Origin	Insertion	Function
Masseter muscle	Zygomatic arch	Lateral surface of mandibular branch from the mandibular notch to the angle of the mandible	Closes the mouth
Temporal muscle	Temporal bone	Apex and medial surface of coronoid process of mandible down to its base	Closes the mouth and pulls back the mandible

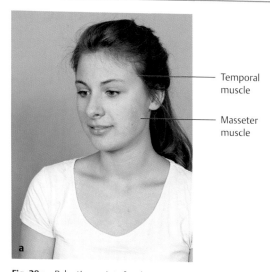

Fig. 28 a   Palpation points for the masseter and temporal muscles.

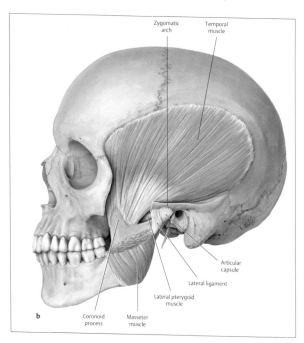

Fig. 28 b
Muscles of
mastication.

■ Lateral Pterygoid Muscle and Medial Pterygoid Muscle (Fig. 29 a)

Muscle	Origin	Insertion	Function
Lateral ptery-goid muscle	Main head: lateral surface of lateral lamina of pterygoid process, maxillary tuberosity. Accessory head: greater wing of sphenoid bone	Pterygoid fovea (condylar process of the mandible), articular disk of temporomandibular joint	Closes the mouth and moves the mandible forward if there is bilateral innervation; side-to-side movements of the jaw if there is only unilateral innervation. Parts of the lateral pterygoid muscle also contribute to opening the mouth
Medial ptery-goid muscle	Pterygoid fossa (sphenoidal bone, pterygoid process). Palatine bone	Medial surface of angle of mandible facing masseter muscle	Grinding movements

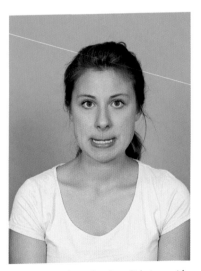

Fig. 29 a   The lateral and medial pterygoid muscle cannot be palpated externally.

Muscles of Facial Expression

All of the muscles of facial expression (**Fig. 29 b**) insert at the margin of the epidermis. As a result, they move the skin and are rarely covered with muscle fascia.

All of these muscles are innervated by branches of the facial nerve (seventh cranial nerve) (**Fig. 29 c**). Nerve damage results in flaccid paralysis of all muscles on the affected side of the face. The mouth sags and the eye no longer closes.

■ Muscles of the Area around the Mouth

Muscle	Origin	Insertion	Function
Levator labii superioris alaeque nasi muscle (**Fig. 30**)	Emerges from the muscle mass of the orbicularis oculi muscle (maxilla, frontal process)	Nostrils and upper lip	Facial expression: movements of the lips and the nostril Cheeks and skin of the chin
Levator labii superioris muscle (**Fig. 30**)	Emerges from the muscle mass of the orbicularis oculi muscle (infra-orbital margin)	Nostrils and upper lip	See levator labii superioris alaeque nasi muscle
Zygomaticus minor muscle (**Fig. 30**)	Emerges from the orbicularis oculi muscle (zygomatic bone, lateral surface)	Corner of the mouth	See levator labii superioris alaeque nasi muscle
Zygomaticus major muscle (**Fig. 31**)	Zygomatic bone, lateral surface	Corner of the mouth	Muscles of facial expression (smiling muscles)
Risorius muscle (usually part of the platysma) (**Fig. 32**)	Masseteric fascia	Corner of the mouth	Pulls back the corner of the mouth

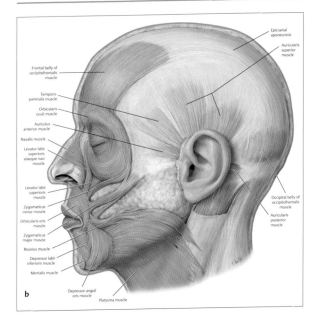

Fig. 29 b
Muscles of facial expression.

Epicranial aponeurosis

Auricularis superior muscle

Frontal belly of occipitofrontalis muscle

Temporo-parietalis muscle

Orbicularis oculi muscle

Auriculus anterior muscle

Nasalis muscle

Levator labii superioris alaeque nasi muscle

Levator labii superioris muscle

Zygomaticus minor muscle

Orbicularis oris muscle

Zygomaticus major muscle

Risorius muscle

Depressor labii inferioris muscle

Mentalis muscle

Occipital belly of occipitofrontalis muscle

Auricularis posterior muscle

b

Depressor anguli oris muscle

Platysma muscle

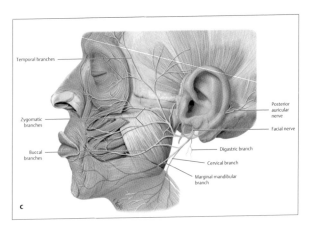

Fig. 29 c
Facial nerve.

Temporal branches

Zygomatic branches

Buccal branches

Posterior auricular nerve

Facial nerve

Digastric branch

Cervical branch

Marginal mandibular branch

c

Muscle	Origin	Insertion	Function
Depressor anguli oris muscle (**Fig. 33**)	Base of mandible	Corner of the mouth and lower lip	Pulls down the corner of the mouth
Levator anguli oris muscle (**Fig. 34**)	Maxilla Canine fossa	Muscles of the upper lip and corner of the mouth	Lifts the corner of the mouth
Depressor labii inferioris muscle (**Fig. 35**)	Base of mandible	Lower lip	Pulls down the lower lip
Orbicularis oris muscle (**Fig. 36**)	Has marginal and labial parts	Oral fissure	Puckers the lips
Mentalis muscle (**Fig. 37**)	Alveolar yoke of lower lateral incisor	Skin of the chin	Pouting muscle
Transversus menti muscle (**Fig. 37**)	Anterior and lateral mandible	Corner of the mouth	See mentalis muscle
Buccinator muscle (**Fig. 38**)	Body of mandible, maxilla, posterior end of alveolar process, bucco-pharyngeal fascia	Corner of the mouth	Narrows the atrium of the oral cavity, presses out air; important for chewing

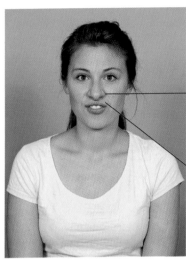

Levator labii superioris muscle and levator labii superioris alaeque nasi muscle

Zygomaticus minor muscle

Fig. 30   Palpation points for the levator labii superioris alaeque nasi muscle, levator labii superioris muscle, and zygomaticus minor muscle.

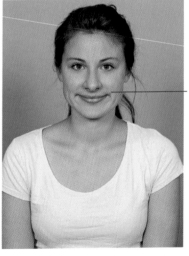

Zygomaticus major muscle

Fig. 31   Palpation point for the zygomaticus major muscle.

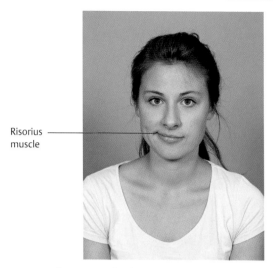

Risorius
muscle

Fig. 32 Palpation point for the risorius muscle.

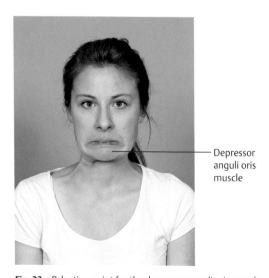

Depressor
anguli oris
muscle

Fig. 33 Palpation point for the depressor anguli oris muscle.

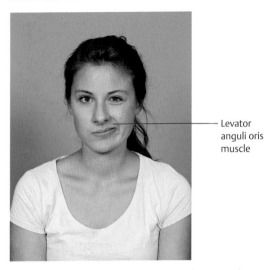

Levator
anguli oris
muscle

Fig. 34   Palpation point for the levator anguli oris muscle.

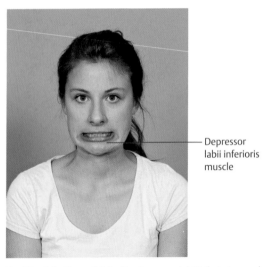

Depressor
labii inferioris
muscle

Fig. 35   Palpation point for the depressor labii inferioris muscle.

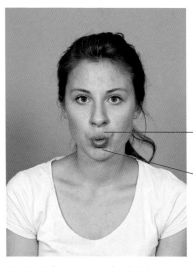

Marginal part of the orbicularis oris muscle

Labial part of the orbicularis oris muscle

Fig. 36 Palpation points for the labial muscle and marginal parts of the orbicularis oris muscle.

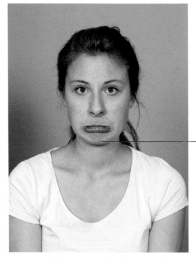

Mentalis muscle and transversus menti muscle

Fig. 37 Palpation point for the mentalis muscle and the transversus menti muscle.

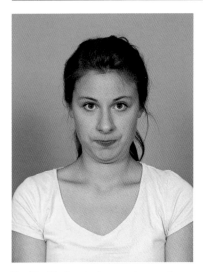

Fig. 38   The buccinator muscle cannot be palpated.

■ Muscles of the Scalp (Epicranius Muscles) (Fig. 39)

Muscle	Origin	Insertion	Function
Occipitofrontalis muscle, frontal belly	Supra-orbital margin	Epicranial aponeurosis	Scalp movements
Occipitofrontalis muscle, occipital belly	Highest nuchal line	Epicranial aponeurosis	Scalp movements
Temporoparietalis muscle	Temporal fascia, superficial layer	Skin and temporal fascia superior to and anterior to the auricle	Scalp movements

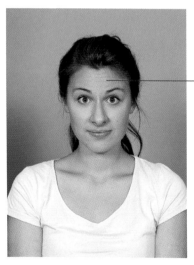

— Epicranial muscles

Fig. 39 Palpation point for the epicranial muscles.

■ Muscles of the Nose

Muscle	Origin	Insertion	Function
Nasalis muscle (**Fig. 40**)			Nostril movements
Transverse part	Area superior to canine root	Aponeurosis on dorsal nose	
Alar part	Area over lateral incisor	Margins of nostrils	
Depressor septi nasi muscle (**Fig. 41**)	Area superior to middle incisor	Nasal cartilaginous septum	Lowers the nostrils

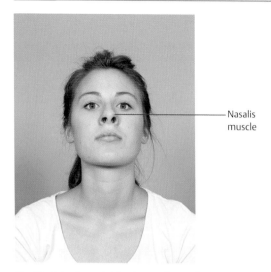

Nasalis muscle

Fig. 40   Palpation point for the nasalis muscle.

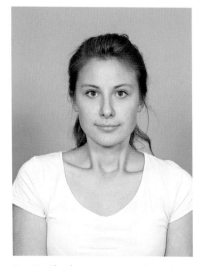

Fig. 41   The depressor septi nasi muscle cannot be palpated.

■ Muscles of the Palpebral Fissure

Muscle	Origin	Insertion	Function
Orbicularis oculi muscle (**Fig. 42**)			
Orbital part	Maxilla, frontal process, medial angle of eye	Surrounds the orbital opening in a sphincter-like manner; partially goes up to the eyebrow	At the external angle of the eye, wrinkles develop in a radial manner. Closes eyelids Compresses the lacrimal sac Moves the eyebrows
Palpebral part	Medial palpebral ligament	Lateral palpebral raphe	
Lacrimal part	Posterior lacrimal crest	Surrounds lacrimal canal and sac	
Depressor supercilii muscle (**Fig. 43**)	Frontal bone, nasal part	Skin of the eyebrow	Acts on the skin of eyebrows and forehead
Corrugator supercilii muscle (**Fig. 43**)	Frontal bone, nasal part	Skin of the eyebrow	Acts on the skin of eyebrows and forehead
Procerus muscle (**Fig. 44**)	Bony dorsal nose	Skin of the glabella	Lifts the skin of the nose

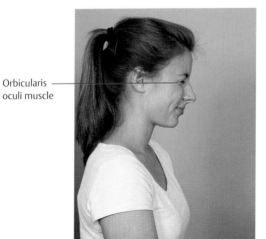

Orbicularis oculi muscle

Fig. 42 Palpation point for the orbicularis oculi muscle.

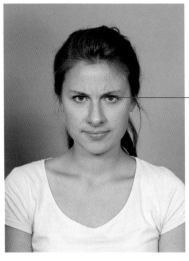

Depressor supercilii muscle and corrugator superciliii muscle

Fig. 43 Palpation point for the depressor supercilii muscle and the corrugator supercilii muscle.

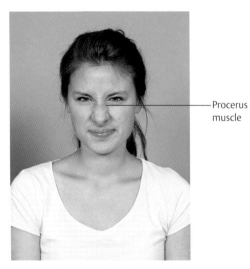

Procerus muscle

Fig. 44 Palpation point for the procerus muscle.

■ Muscles of the Outer Ear

Muscle	Origin	Insertion	Function
Auricularis anterior muscle	Temporal fascia, superficial layer	Spine of helix	Movements of the auricle
Auricularis superior muscle	Epicranial aponeurosis	Root of auricle	Movements of the auricle
Auricularis posterior muscle	Mastoid process, tendon of sternocleido-mastoid muscle	Root of auricle	Movements of the auricle

For the sake of completeness, the muscles of the outer ear are listed here. They are also considered muscles of facial expression. In practice, however, they do not play a significant role for muscle testing since they can rarely be used actively.

■ Platysma Muscle

The platysma muscle is a flat superficial muscle in the neck that directly inserts into the skin. Its trajectory begins at the corner of the mouth, widens greatly across the neck and clavicle, and ends at the skin on the chest at the second rib. The platysma muscle is also considered to be a muscle of facial expression.

- Innervation: facial nerve
- Function: tightens the skin in the neck area

■ Muscles of the Eye (Figs. 45 and 46)

Since these muscles are situated in the orbital cavity and cannot be palpated, their origins and insertions are not described here.

Muscle	Function
Superior rectus muscle Oculomotor nerve	Lifts the eye and rolls it inward
Inferior rectus muscle Oculomotor nerve	Lowers the eye and rolls it outward
Lateral rectus muscle Abducens nerve	Brings about an outward movement of the eye (abduction)
Medial rectus muscle Oculomotor nerve	Brings about an inward movement of the eye toward the nose (adduction)
Superior oblique muscle Trochlear nerve	Lowers the eye and rolls it inward
Inferior oblique muscle Oculomotor nerve	Lifts the eye and rolls it outward
Levator palpebrae superioris muscle Oculomotor nerve	Lifts the eyelid, facial expression of surprise

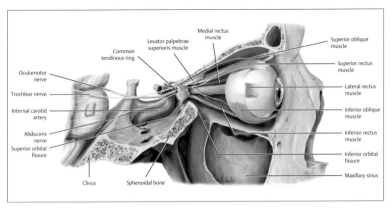

Fig. 45   Muscles of the eye.

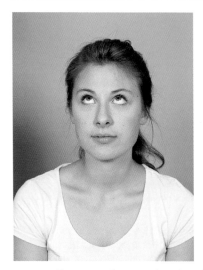

Fig. 46 a   The eye muscles cannot be palpated.

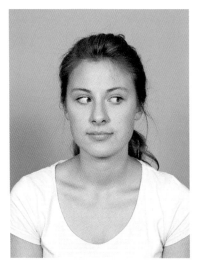

Fig. 46 b   The eye muscles cannot be palpated.

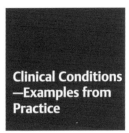

Clinical Conditions —Examples from Practice

Facial Nerve Palsy (Seventh Cranial Nerve)

Facial nerve palsy manifests itself as weakness or complete paralysis of the muscles of facial expression on the affected side of the face. It is characterized by a sagging mouth and an inability to close the mouth completely. Patients are unable to wrinkle their forehead and cannot close their eye completely on the affected side. Symptoms are most pronounced when the patient attempts to laugh or speak.

In most cases, the condition is referred to as idiopathic facial nerve palsy. It is usually caused by damage to the facial nerve (seventh cranial nerve).

■ (Herpes) Virus Infection

Various pathogens, viruses (especially herpes viruses) as well as bacteria, can trigger facial nerve palsy.

■ Other Factors

Facial nerve palsy can also be caused by pressure-induced damage to the nerve, owing to tumors, edema, bleeding, or congenital deformities, although this is rare.

Facial nerve injury can also lead to paralysis of the platysma muscle.

Abducens Nerve Palsy (Sixth Cranial Nerve)

Affected patients gaze inward and are unable to look sideways with the damaged eye, which results in the head position characteristic of this condition. Patients turn their head to the affected side.

The nerve's unique path causes it to become damaged when intracranial pressure is elevated.

 Trochlear Nerve Palsy (Fourth Cranial Nerve)

Patients experience double vision when reading and climbing stairs. To compensate, they tilt their head away from the affected side. Damage to the trochlear nerve is often the result of head injury.

 Oculomotor Nerve Palsy (Third Cranial Nerve)

When the oculomotor nerve is damaged, the superior and inferior rectus muscles, medial rectus muscle, inferior oblique muscle, and levator palpebrae superioris muscle are paralyzed. This results in a down and out position in the affected eye, with the eyelid drooping over the pupil (ptosis).

4
Spine

**Muscles and
Manual Muscle
Testing of
the Spine**

Extension of the Cervical, Thoracic, and Lumbar Spine (Figs. 47 and 48)

	Muscle	Origin	Insertion
	Erector spinae muscle, lateral tract		
	Intertransversarii muscles		
1A	*Iliocostalis lumborum muscle*	Sacrum, outer lip of iliac crest, thoracolumbar fascia	Costal processes of upper lumbar vertebrae, lower sixth to ninth ribs
1B	*Iliocostalis thoracis muscle*	Lower six ribs	Upper six ribs
1C	*Iliocostalis cervicis muscle*	Sixth to third rib	Transverse processes of C6–C4 vertebrae
	(Dorsal rami of C4–L3)		
2A	*Longissimus thoracis muscle*	Sacrum, spinous processes of lumbar vertebrae, transverse processes of lower thoracic vertebrae	Medial: accessory processes of lumbar vertebrae, transverse processes of thoracic vertebrae. Lateral: ribs, costal processes of lumbar vertebrae, thoracolumbar fascia
2B	*Longissimus cervicis muscle*	Transverse processes of T1–T6 vertebrae	Posterior tubercles of transverse processes of C2–C5 vertebrae
2C	*Longissimus capitis muscle*	Transverse processes of T3–T5 vertebrae and C5–C7 vertebrae	Mastoid process
	(Dorsal rami of C2–L5)		

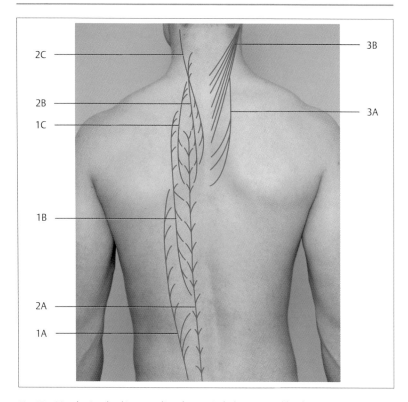

Fig. 47   Muscles involved in extending the cervical, thoracic, and lumbar spine:
1A   Iliocostalis lumborum muscle
1B   Iliocostalis thoracis muscle
1C   Iliocostalis cervicis muscle
2A   Longissimus thoracis muscle
2B   Longissimus cervicis muscle
2C   Longissimus capitis muscle
3A   Splenius cervicis muscle
3B   Splenius capitis muscle

	Muscle	Origin	Insertion
	Spinotransversales muscles		
3A	*Splenius cervicis muscle*	Spinous processes of T(3)4–T(5)6 and C4–C7 vertebrae	Transverse processes of C1 and C2 vertebrae
3B	*Splenius capitis muscle*	Spinous processes of T1–T3 and C4–C7 vertebrae	Area of the mastoid process
	(Dorsal rami of C1–C8)		
	Medial tract		
	Rectus muscles		
4A	*Interspinales lumborum muscles*	Arranged in a segmental fashion in cervical and lumbar spine and between T1	
4B	*Interspinales thoracis muscles*	and T2 and between T2 and T3 vertebrae, and between	
4C	*Interspinales cervicis muscles*	T11 and T12 vertebrae and between T12 and L1 vertebrae; they connect the adjacent spinous processes	
	(Dorsal rami of C1–T3 and T11–L5)		
5A	*Posterior cervical intertransversarii muscles*	Connect the adjacent posterior tubercles of the transverse processes of C2–C7 vertebrae	
	(Dorsal rami of C1–C6)		
5B	*Medial lumbar intertransversarii muscles*	Connect the mammillary and accessory processes of the adjacent lumbar vertebrae	
	(Dorsal rami of L1–L4)		

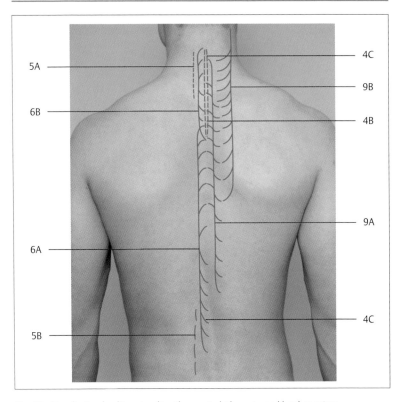

Fig. 48   Muscles involved in extending the cervical, thoracic, and lumbar spine:
4A   Interspinales lumborum muscles
4B   Interspinales thoracis muscles
4C   Interspinales cervicis muscles
5A   Posterior cervical intertransversarii muscles
5B   Medial lumbar intertransversarii muscles
6A   Spinalis thoracis muscle
6B   Spinalis cervicis muscle
9A   Semispinalis thoracis and cervicis muscle
9B   Semispinalis capitis muscle

	Muscle	Origin	Insertion
6A	*Spinalis thoracis muscle*	Spinous processes of L3–T10 vertebrae	Spinous processes of T8–T2 vertebrae
6B	*Spinalis cervicis muscle*	Spinous processes of T2–C6 vertebrae	Spinous processes of C4–C2 vertebrae
	(Dorsal rami of C2–T10)		
	Oblique muscles		
7A	*Rotatores (cervicis) brevis and longi muscles*		
7B	*Longissimus thoracis (and lumborum) muscle*	In the thorax in particular, these muscles originate from the transverse processes and insert at the next higher spinous process or skip the next spinous process and insert at their base	
	(Dorsal rami of T1–T11)		
8	*Multifidus muscle*	Superficial leaf of fascia of longissimus muscle, dorsal surface of sacrum, mammillary processes of lumbar vertebrae, transverse processes of thoracic vertebrae, articular processes of C7–C4 vertebrae	Muscle bundles skip over two to four vertebrae and insert at the spinous processes of the respective next higher vertebrae
	(Dorsal rami of C1–S4)		
9A	*Semispinalis thoracis and cervicis muscles*	Transverse processes of all thoracic vertebrae	Spinous processes of T1–T6 and C4–C7 vertebrae
9B	*Semispinalis capitis muscle*	Transverse processes of T4–T7 vertebrae, articular processes of C3–C7 vertebrae	Between the superior and inferior nuchal line
	(Dorsal rami of T4–T6, C3–C6, and C1–C5)		

■ Extension of the Cervical Spine (Fig. 49)

	Muscle	Origin	Insertion
	Short neck muscles		
10	*Rectus capitis posterior minor muscle* (Suboccipital nerve C1)	Posterior tubercle of atlas	Medial area of inferior nuchal line
11	*Rectus capitis posterior major muscle* (Suboccipital nerve C1)	Spinous process of C2 vertebra	Inferior nuchal line
12	*Obliquus capitis superior muscle* (Suboccipital nerve C1)	Atlantic transverse process	Occipital bone
13	*Obliquus capitis inferior muscle* (Suboccipital nerve C1)	Spinous process of C2 vertebra	Atlantic transverse process

Clinical Symptoms

Shortening: Results in restricted range of motion in the direction of flexion, lateral bending, and rotation of the cervical spine. Since the short neck muscles are also affected, inclination of the atlanto-occipital joint is also restricted. Increased extension of the upper and mid-cervical spine usually results in an abnormal position of the other vertebral segments, owing to compensation. The range of motion of these segments can be highly restricted.

Unilateral contractures lead to a scoliotic posture and functional disturbances in the motion of cervical spine segments. Pain radiating into the shoulder and arm, as well as headache or dizziness, may be the result of persistent muscle shortening.

Weakness: If the cervical spine extensors are weak, the patient will have insufficient head control and possibly altered balance.

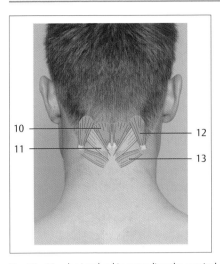

Fig. 49   Muscles involved in extending the cervical spine that cannot be palpated:
10   Rectus capitis posterior minor muscle
11   Rectus capitis posterior major muscle
12   Obliquus capitis superior muscle
13   Obliquus capitis inferior muscle

1. Cervical spine extensors are palpated with the patient lying on one side. The examiner places a pillow under the patient's head to prevent the cervical spine from tilting to the side.

   The short neck muscles can be palpated only as a unit. The other cervical spine extensors can also be evaluated only as a unit.

2. The patient lies on one side (**Fig. 50a**). The examiner stabilizes the shoulder girdle. Full range of motion consists of cervical spine extension and a backward movement in the atlanto-occipital joint.

3. The patient lies prone (**Fig. 50b**). The patient's head hangs over the end of the table and the examiner stabilizes the upper thoracic spine. The range of motion is tested as described for an evaluation of grade 2 muscle strength.

4. 5. 6. Starting position, stabilization, and range of motion as for grade 3 (**Fig. 50c**).

   The examiner applies resistance to the back of the patient's head. The range of motion is tested as described for an evaluation of grade 2 muscle strength.

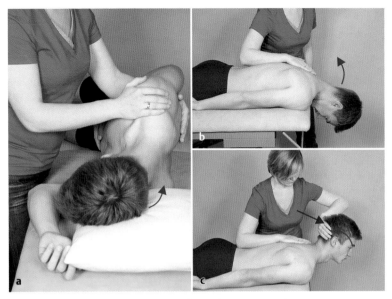

Fig. 50 Testing of cervical spine extension for grades 2, 3, 4, 5, and 6.

■ Extension of the Thoracic Spine

> ### Clinical Symptoms
>
> **Shortening:** Restricted range of motion for flexion, rotation, and lateral bending of the thoracic spine.
>
> Unilateral shortening leads to a scoliotic posture of the spine and functional disturbances in the motion of the thoracic spine segments.
>
> This may result in pain radiating into the shoulder and arm.
>
> **Weakness:** Weakness of the thoracic spine extensors is primarily manifested by an inability to straighten the thoracic spine. Thoracic kyphosis is increased and the adjacent vertebral segments also exhibit an exaggerated physiological curvature (see pp. 112–116).

[1] The examiner palpates the thoracic spine extensors with the patient lying prone. The patient is asked to raise his or her head, to allow the examiner to palpate paravertebral tension. The thoracic spine extensors cannot be palpated separately and the deeper muscles cannot be palpated at all (see **Figs. 47** and **48**).

[2] The patient moves into a kneeling position, with the head lowered and the arms at the sides (**Fig. 51 a**). In this position, the lumbar spine extensors for the most part are not active. The arms are next to the body. The examiner stabilizes the pelvis and the lumbar spine.
The patient is asked to raise the head, shoulder girdle, and arms. The patient partially extends the thoracic spine.

[3] Starting position and stabilization as for evaluation of grade 2 muscle strength. The patient fully extends the thoracic spine.

[4] Starting position, stabilization, and range of motion as for grade 3 (**Fig. 51 b**). However, the patient holds the arms in the shape of a goalpost (higher level of difficulty because of the longer lever arm).

[5][6] Starting position, stabilization, and range of motion as for grade 3. The patient now clasps the arms behind the head (**Fig. 51 c**).

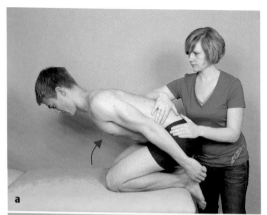

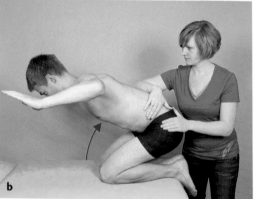

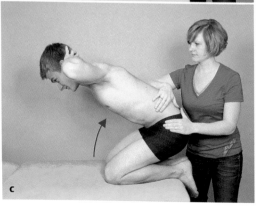

Fig. 51 Testing of thoracic spine extension for grades 2, 3, 4, 5, and 6.

■ **Extension of the Lumbar Spine**

Clinical Symptoms

Shortening: Restricted range of motion in the direction of flexion, rotation, and lateral bending of the spine. This restriction increases the lordotic curvature of the lumbar spine, which leads to increased pelvic tilt, more pronounced hip flexion and, in many cases, weakening of the abdominal muscles and hip joint extensors. Unilateral contractures can cause scoliotic postures and functional disturbances in the lumbar, pelvic, and hip regions.

Weakness: Weakness of the lumbar spine extensors may be manifested as a kyphotic posture when the patient is sitting, or as lumbar spine kyphosis when the patient lifts objects from the ground. Affected patients may report symptoms associated with lumbar hypermobility in their history, such as a feeling of instability and experiencing pain when they stand for longer periods, with movement relieving this pain. Patients may also report night pain relieved by movement. In most cases, muscle strengthening training is very successful.

[1] The examiner palpates the lumbar spine extensors, with the patient lying prone.
The patient is asked to raise the head and thorax. The examiner palpates the involved muscles together. The deep extensors of the lumbar spine cannot be palpated (**Figs. 47** and **48**).

[2] The patient lies on one side at the edge of the table (**Fig. 52 a**). The hip and knee joints are flexed at 90° and the lumbar spine is placed in kyphosis.
The examiner holds the weight of the patient's legs and stabilizes the upper body. The patient is asked to extend the lumbar spine by moving the pelvis dorsally. During this movement, the hip and knee joints remain flexed at 90°.

[3] The patient lies prone (**Fig. 52 b**). The pelvis and legs hang over the end of the table, so that the lumbar spine is placed in kyphosis. The knee and hip joints are flexed at 90° and the examiner holds the lower legs. The patient initiates extension of the lumbar spine from the pelvis. The knee and hip joints remain flexed at 90°.

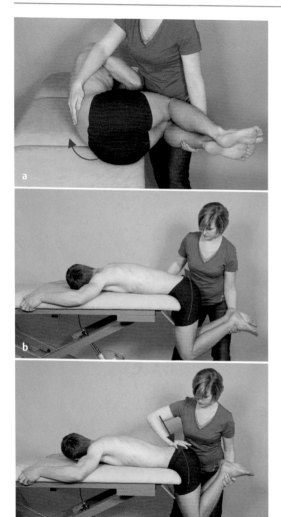

Fig. 52 Testing of lumbar spine extension for grades 2, 3, 4, 5, and 6.

4 5 6 Starting position as for grade 3 muscle testing (**Fig. 52 c**). The examiner applies resistance on the sacrum.

Flexion of the Cervical Spine (Fig. 53)

Muscle	Origin	Insertion
Rectus capitis anterior muscle C1 cervical plexus	Lateral mass of atlas	Basilar part (occipital bone)
Longus capitis muscle Cervical plexus (C1–C4)	Anterior tubercles of transverse processes of C3–C6 vertebrae	Basilar part (occipital bone)
Longus colli muscle		
Lateral superior fibers	Anterior tubercles of transverse processes of C5–C2 vertebrae	Anterior tubercle of anterior atlas
Lateral inferior fibers	T1–T3 vertebral bodies	Anterior tubercle of C6 vertebra
Medial fibers Cervical and brachial plexus (C2–C8)	Upper thoracic and lower cervical vertebral bodies	Upper cervical vertebral bodies
Rectus capitis lateralis muscle (C1)	Transverse process of atlas	Jugular process of occipital bone
Anterior cervical intertransversarii muscles *Branch from dorsal ramus of spinal nerve (C2–C6)* Anterior branches (C2–C6)	Six small bundles between anterior tubercles of transverse processes of cervical spine	
1 *Sternocleidomastoid muscle* Accessory nerve and fibers from C1–C2	Sternum, clavicle	Mastoid process, superior nuchal line

Muscle	Origin	Insertion
Scalenus anterior muscle Brachial plexus (C5–C7)	Anterior tubercles of transverse processes of C(3)4–C6 vertebrae	First rib
Scalenus medius muscle Cervical and brachial plexus (C4–C8)	Posterior tubercles of transverse processes of C(1)2–C7 vertebrae	First rib First intercostal space
Scalenus posterior muscle Brachial plexus (C7–C8)	Posterior tubercles of transverse processes of C5–C7 vertebrae	Second (third) rib

Infrahyoid Muscles (Innervation: Anterior Branches of the Cervical Plexus C1–C3 (Ansa Cervicalis Profundus)

Muscle	Origin	Insertion
Sternohyoid muscle	Posterior surface of manubrium of sternum, possibly the sternal end of clavicle	Posterior surface of hyoid bone
Omohyoid muscle	Body of hyoid bone	Superior border of scapula
Sternothyroid muscle	Posterior surface of manubrium of sternum	Thyroid cartilage
Thyrohyoid muscle	Oblique line of thyroid cartilage	Hyoid bone

Clinical Symptoms

Shortening: The deep flexors of the cervical spine are usually very weak and in a stretched position. Only the sternocleidomastoid muscles tend to shorten, which extends the atlanto-occipital joint and increases the lordotic curvature of the mid-cervical spine (see pp. 115 and 116).

The sternocleidomastoid muscles can only flex the cervical spine if the deep flexors place the atlanto-occipital joint in flexion and maintain this position. If the muscles are shortened on only one side, the patient will have a twisted neck. In this case, the patient's head tilts toward the affected side and is turned toward the non-affected side.

Shortening of the scalenus muscles also increases the lordotic curvature. If these muscles shorten unilaterally, lateral bending toward the non-affected side is usually restricted.

Weakness: Unilateral weakness of the sternocleidomastoid muscle also causes a twisted neck. In this case, the patient's head tilts toward the non-affected side and is turned toward the affected side.

If the deeper cervical spine flexors are weakened, the patient cannot adequately perform a forward nodding movement.

The atlanto-occipital joint cannot be placed in flexion and the sternocleidomastoid muscles cannot create flexion, owing to the altered course of the axis of motion. Their function is inverted and they act as extensors. This process is particularly apparent when the patient is told to lift his or her head while lying supine. The atlanto-occipital joint cannot be flexed. The head is raised with the cervical spine in extension.

The weakness of the deep flexors causes the extensors to predominate, which causes the atlanto-occipital joint to hyperextend. This may result in headaches.

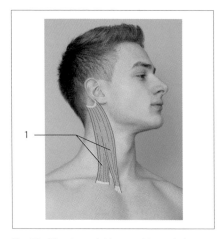

Fig. 53 The sternocleidomastoid muscle is involved in flexion of the cervical spine.
1 Sternocleidomastoid muscle

1. The examiner palpates the cervical spine flexors with the patient supine.
   Only the sternocleidomastoid and scalenus muscles can be palpated. The deeper flexors of the cervical spine cannot be palpated because they are covered by these muscles.
2. The patient is supine (**Fig. 54a**). The patient's head hangs over the edge of the table and is held by the examiner. The patient partially flexes the cervical spine.
3. Starting position as for evaluation of grade 2 muscle strength (**Fig. 54b**). The movement is executed fully. Before the patient flexes the cervical spine, a forward nodding motion must be performed in the atlanto-occipital joint.
4. 5. 6. Starting position as for grade 2 (**Fig. 54c**). The examiner applies resistance to the patient's forehead and chin.

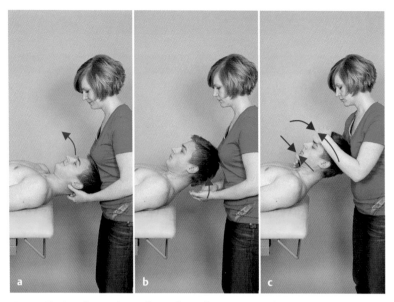

Fig. 54   Testing of cervical spine flexion for grades 2, 3, 4, 5, and 6.

Flexion of the Trunk (Fig. 55)

	Muscle	Origin	Insertion
1	*Rectus abdominis muscle*	External surface of cartilage of fifth to seventh ribs, xyphoid process	Pubic crest
	Intercostal nerves (T5–T12)		
2	*External oblique muscle*	Arises with eight digitations from external surfaces of fifth to twelfth ribs	Outer lip of iliac crest, aponeurosis of ilio-inguinal ligament
	Intercostal nerves (T5–T12)		
	Internal oblique muscle	Iliac crest, deep leaf of thoracolumbar fascia, anterior superior iliac spine	Lower borders of the three lower ribs, medial in the aponeurosis, ilio-inguinal ligament
	Intercostal nerves (T5–T12)		
	Transversus abdominis muscle	With six digitations from the inner surface of the cartilage of seventh to twelfth ribs, deep leaf of thoracolumbar fascia, internal lip of iliac crest, anterior superior iliac spine, inguinal ligament	Aponeurosis, ilio-inguinal ligament
	Intercostal nerves (T7–T12, L1)		

Clinical Symptoms

Shortening: Tension on the shortened trunk flexors makes it nearly impossible for the patient to straighten the spine into its physiological curvatures.

The pelvis is tilted dorsally and at the pubic bone where the rectus abdominis muscle inserts. This may result in pain syndromes.

The lumbar spine cannot be placed sufficiently in lordosis and the thoracic spine has an exaggerated kyphotic curvature. This influences the

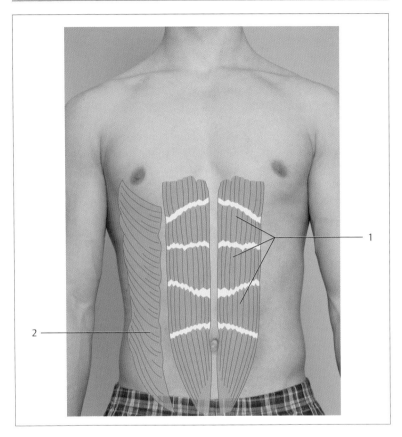

Fig. 55   Muscles involved in trunk flexion:
1   Rectus abdominis muscle
2   External oblique muscle

position of the shoulder girdle and cervical spine. If these deviations persist, they will cause muscle imbalances in the shoulder girdle and neck (see p. 116).

Weakness: Patients with this kind of weakness can sit up from a supine position only if they support themselves with their arms.

The lumbar spine has a hyperlordotic curvature and the pelvis is tilted.

If the abdominal muscles are not innervated, or only minimally innervated, respiratory volume is reduced.

☐1 The examiner palpates the trunk flexors with the patient supine and the knees bent. The internal oblique muscle and the transversus abdominis muscle are covered by the external oblique muscle.
Contraction of the abdominal muscles can be felt when the patient coughs, laughs, or lifts the head. If the abdominal muscles vary in strength or innervation, the umbilicus will shift toward the stronger part.

☐2 The patient is supine, with the knees bent (**Fig. 56 a**). The arms are next to the body. The patient is asked to raise the head, arms, shoulder blades, and upper thoracic spine off the table.

☐3 Starting position as for grade 2. The patient lifts the entire thoracic spine off the table.

☐4 Starting position as for grade 2 (**Fig. 56 b**). With the arms folded in front of the chest, the patient lifts the entire thoracic spine off the table.

☐5☐6 Starting position as for grade 2 (**Fig. 56 c**). With the hands clasped behind the head, the patient lifts the entire thoracic spine off the table.

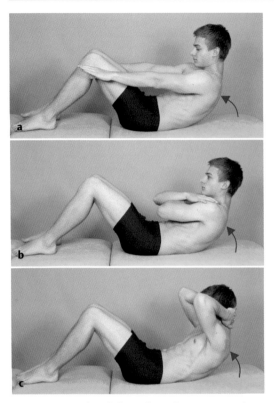

Fig. 56   Testing of trunk flexion for grades 2, 3, 4, 5, and 6.

Rotation of the Trunk (Fig. 57)

	Muscle	Origin	Insertion
1	*External oblique muscle*	Arises with eight digitations from external surfaces of fifth to twelfth ribs	Outer lip of iliac crest, aponeurosis
	Intercostal nerves (T5–T12)		
	Internal oblique muscle	Iliac crest, deep leaf of thoracolumbar fascia, anterior superior iliac spine	Lower borders of the three lower ribs, medial in aponeurosis
	Intercostal nerves (T5–T12)		

Clinical Symptoms

Shortening: Unilateral shortening of the short rotators leads to functional disturbances in the motion of individual spine segments and causes scoliotic posture. This is exacerbated by unilateral shortening of the abdominal oblique muscles. Rotation in the individual spine segments is very important for physiological gait. During the various gait phases, these segments rotate in a clockwise and counterclockwise fashion, to compensate for each other. If this rotation is restricted by muscular shortening, pronounced changes in gait can be observed.

Weakness: Weakness in the trunk rotators is primarily manifested in the gait pattern.

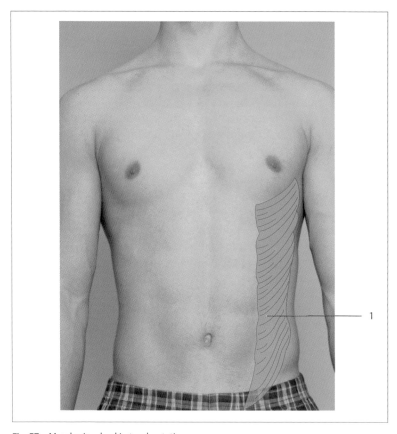

Fig. 57 Muscles involved in trunk rotation:
1   External oblique muscle

[1] The examiner palpates the external oblique muscle with the patient supine.

Muscle contraction can be felt when the patient coughs, laughs, or lifts the head. If the muscle varies in strength or innervation, the umbilicus will shift toward the stronger part during contraction. The oblique spinal extensors act in a rotating fashion if they are only unilaterally innervated. These muscles cannot be palpated because the rotator muscles and multifidus muscles are the deepest layer of the back muscles.

[2] The patient is supine, with the knees bent (**Fig. 58 a**). The examiner stabilizes the pelvis.

When rotating to the right, the patient places the left hand on the right shoulder. The patient lifts the left side of the thorax partially and turns it toward the right side.

[3] Starting position and stabilization as for grade 2. The patient lifts the corresponding side of the thorax completely, that is, down to the lower costal arch, off the table and turns to the opposite side.

[4] [5] [6] Starting position and stabilization as for grade 2. The movement is performed as described for grade 3.

The examiner applies resistance to the patient's shoulder (**Fig. 58 b**).

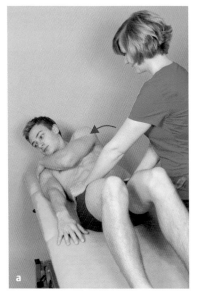
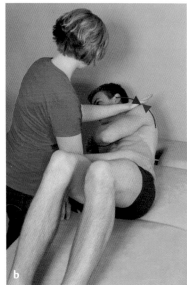

Fig. 58 Testing of trunk rotation for grades 2, 3, 4, 5, and 6.
a Test for grade 2.
b The examiner applies resistance to the shoulder.

Lateral Bending of the Trunk (Figs. 59 and 60)

	Muscle
1	Erector spinae muscle (see p. 109)
	Lateral tract, transverse muscles
	Iliocostalis lumborum muscle
	Iliocostalis thoracis muscle
	Iliocostalis cervicis muscle
	Longissimus thoracis muscle
	Longissimus cervicis muscle
	Longissimus capitis muscle
	Medial tract/rectus muscles of the spinal extensors
	Interspinales lumborum muscles
	Interspinales thoracis muscles
	Interspinales cervicis muscles
	Thoracic intertransvarsarii muscles
	Posterior cervical intertransversarii muscles
2	*External oblique muscle (see pp. 102 and 103)*
3	*Internal oblique muscle (see p. 102)*
4	*Rectus abdominis muscle (see pp. 98 and 99)*
5	*Latissimus dorsi muscle (see pp. 138 and 139)*
	Quadratus lumborum muscle

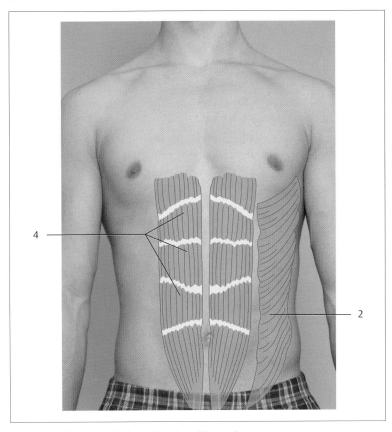

Fig. 59 Muscles involved in lateral bending of the trunk:
2   External oblique muscle
4   Rectus abdominis muscle

Clinical Symptoms

Shortening: Unilateral shortening of the lateral trunk flexors leads to restricted rotation of the trunk, lateral tilt toward the opposite side, and scoliotic posture of the spine.

Functional disturbances may occur in motion of the spinal segment and the lumbar, pelvic, and hip regions.

Weakness: Weakness of the lateral trunk flexors causes muscle-related instability of the trunk and scoliotic posture.

The patient's ability to maintain his or her balance when sitting or standing is diminished.

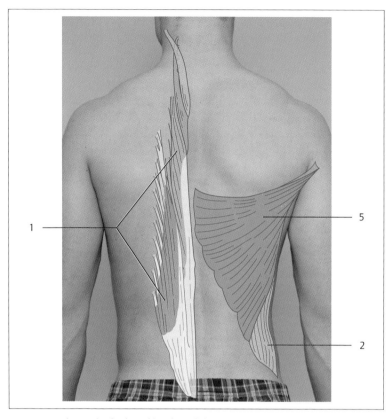

Fig. 60   Muscles involved in lateral bending of the trunk:
1   Erector spinae muscle
2   External oblique muscle
5   Latissimus dorsi muscle

[1] The examiner palpates the involved muscles with the patient lying on one side. The examiner palpates the entire erector spinae muscle.

The deep quadratus lumborum muscle is covered by other muscles, which prevents it from being palpated separately.

[2] The patient is supine, with the upper body on a towel. The examiner stabilizes the pelvis (**Fig. 61 a**). The patient initiates the movement by attempting to touch the knee on the same side with the hand.

[3] The patient lies on one side. The examiner places a pillow under the patient's pelvis, to increase the range of motion (**Fig. 61 b**). The examiner stabilizes the legs and pelvis. The patient's upper arm is extended on the side of the body, while the lower arm is flexed and the hand grasps the top shoulder.

The patient raises the upper body, including the upper lumbar spine.

[4] Starting position, stabilization, and range of motion as for grade 3 (**Fig. 61 c**). The patient's arms are folded in front of the chest for this test.

[5][6] Starting position, stabilization, and range of motion as for grade 3 (**Fig. 61 d**).

For this test, the patient's hands are clasped behind the head.

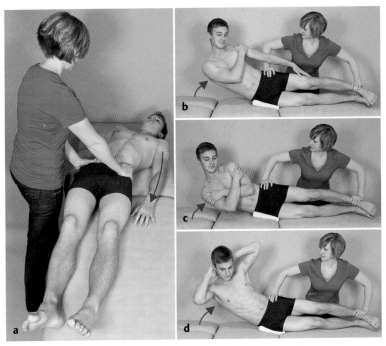

Fig. 61 Testing of lateral bending of the trunk for grades 2, 3, 4, 5, and 6.

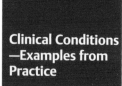

Clinical Conditions —Examples from Practice

Muscle Imbalance of the Trunk

The shape and extent of the sagittal spinal curvature are largely determined by the position of the pelvis. The rotational axis around which the pelvis tilts forward and backward runs through both hip joints. Muscles that directly influence this motion must cross this rotational axis. Since the flexor and extensor muscles of the hip joint cross this rotational axis, their activity and their extensibility are key determinants of the position of the pelvis. As a consequence, the trunk muscles can only influence the position of the pelvis indirectly, and when fixed and mobile attachments are reversed, such as when the upper body is stabilized.

If a person standing upright is viewed from the side, the body's gravity line precisely meets this pelvis rotational axis to tilt and straighten the pelvis. In this case, the pelvis is held in unstable equilibrium; the muscles only need to perform minimal work to maintain balance, and the passive structures (e.g., iliofemoral ligament) are not placed under any pressure (**Fig. 62**).

When this gravity line shifts in front of or behind the hip joint's rotational axis, the muscles immediately respond by increasing their activity. If the upper body is bent forward, the pelvis is tilted and the extensors of the hip joint have to perform more work to keep a person balanced. When the upper body is bent backward, the pelvis is straightened and the activity in the flexors of the hip joint increases (**Fig. 63**).

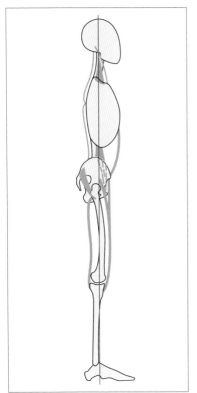

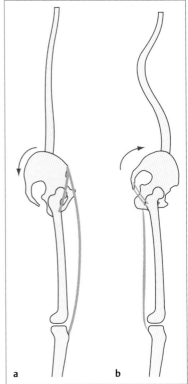

Fig. 62 Trajectory of the gravity line in a person standing upright.

Fig. 63 Change in muscle strength caused by a shift in the gravity line.

The pelvis is stabilized by the muscles acting from the head and, as a result, provides a base for the spine. The muscles running from the pelvis toward the head have little impact if this base is not stable enough. This means that the thigh muscles must first stabilize the pelvis enough for the trunk muscles to unleash their full strength and action. By the same token, the muscles of the lower leg also have to tightly connect the foot and thigh in order for the thigh muscles to perform their work.

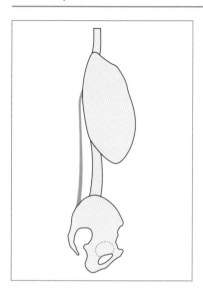

Fig. 64 Lifting effect of the erector spinae muscle on the lower part of the thorax.

Contracting the erector spinae muscle puts the lower segments of the spine in lordosis up to T5–T6, and lifts the lower part of the thorax at the same time (**Fig. 64**). Normal strength and extensibility of the abdominal muscles is required to help stabilize the trunk in this position.

The muscles from the back of the head to the T6 vertebra place this area in lordosis and lift the upper part of the thorax. The more the anterior neck muscles prevent excessive lordosis of the cervical spine, the stronger the lifting movement of the thorax will be (**Fig. 65**).

The spinal extensors in the mid-thoracic spine, which are not as strongly developed, play only a minor role in lifting the spine and thorax.

The sternocleidomastoid muscles also lift the thorax if the cervical spine and head are immobilized. The pectoralis major and pectoralis minor muscles can also be used to lift the thorax if the trapezius and rhomboid muscles pull the scapula toward the spine and hold it in this position (**Fig. 66**).

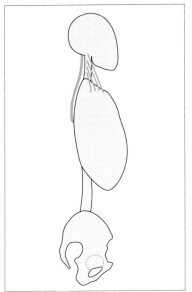

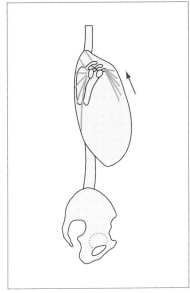

Fig. 65 The upper part of the thorax is lifted by the upper back extensors and the anterior cervical muscles.

Fig. 66 Interaction of the pectoralis major, pectoralis minor, and scapula muscles during lifting of the upper thorax.

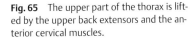

The position and curvature of the cervical spine are primarily dependent on body position. In an upright position, the cervical spine is nearly extended and the head's gravity line is close to that of the vertebral bodies. In a kyphotic posture, the cervical spine compensates through stronger lordosis, and the gravity line moves posterior to the vertebral body. The weight of the head has an even stronger lordotic effect (**Fig. 67**).

The aforementioned description demonstrates that posture involves a fine-tuned interaction between agonists and antagonists with respect to strength and extensibility.

If this muscle balance is disturbed by contractures or muscle weaknesses, deviations occur that not only affect an area in isolation but usually also affect the entire posture. Weakness of agonist muscles often causes contractures in the antagonists. Weakness of the hip joint exten-

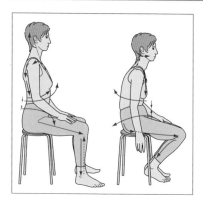

Fig. 67   Cervical spine with straight or kyphotic posture.

sors often occurs in combination with contracture of the hip joint flexors. This shortening, in turn, acts on the spine by increasing lumbar lordosis. Imbalances in the shoulder girdle muscles also lead to changes in the spine's physiological curvature. A typical example is weakness of the rhomboid trapezius muscles combined with contracture of the pectoralis major and pectoralis minor muscles; this is generally characterized by exaggerated kyphosis in the thoracic spine and increased compensatory lordosis in the cervical spine. If the altered position of the cervical spine persists for a long time, it will, in turn, alter the balance between the flexors and extensors of the cervical spine. The posterior neck muscles will become shortened and the anterior muscles weaker. Since the short neck extensors are also contracted, the atlanto-occipital joint is hyperextended.

Of course, posture is also determined by a person's mood or exercise habits. People who are successful and happy are more likely to present themselves with a proud, upright body position, while downtrodden, less successful individuals will tend to have a hunched posture. High-intensity sports such as rowing or cycling, and poor posture at one's desk, can also have a negative impact on posture if they are not counteracted. If they go untreated, these impacts can also lead to muscle imbalances.

5
Upper Extremity

Muscles and Manual Muscle Testing of the Upper Extremity

Scapula

For practical reasons, movements of the shoulder girdle should be separated from those of the shoulder joint during the examination. Of course this is not possible from a purely functional perspective. Shoulder joint movements—in all six degrees of freedom—cannot be executed in a full range of motion and with maximum strength without accompanying movements of the scapula to stabilize it on the thorax.

For this reason, when shoulder mobility is impaired, the strength and range of motion of the shoulder girdle (scapular) movements must always be evaluated.

Conversely, when the strength of the shoulder girdle movements is reduced, shoulder mobility and strength will likely be reduced as well.

■ Elevation of the Scapula (Fig. 68)

	Muscle	Origin	Insertion
1	*Trapezius muscle*		
	Descending (superior) part	Superior nuchal line, external occipital protuberance, ligamentum nuchae	Lateral third of the clavicle
	Transverse (middle) part	Spinal processes of C7–T3 vertebrae, supraspinal ligaments	Acromial end of clavicle, acromion, scapular spine
	Accessory nerve and ramus trapezius (C2–C4)		

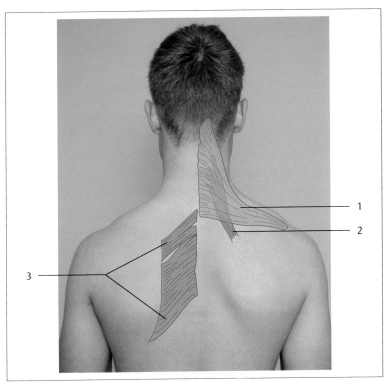

Fig. 68 Muscles involved in elevating the scapula:
1   Trapezius muscle
2   Levator scapulae muscle
3   Rhomboid muscles

	Muscle	Origin	Insertion
2	*Levator scapulae muscle*	Transverse processes of C1–C4 vertebrae	Superior angle of scapula
	Dorsal scapular nerve (C4–C5)		
3	*Rhomboid muscles*	Spinal processes of C6–C7 vertebrae, spinal processes of T1–T4 vertebrae	Medial border of scapula
	Dorsal scapular nerve (C4–C5)		

Clinical Symptoms

Shortening: The scapula is elevated. Cervical spine mobility is restricted in terms of lateral bending, rotation, and flexion.

In the glenohumeral joint, shortening of these muscles hampers the patient from raising his or her shoulder, since the required scapula rotation (with the inferior angle of the scapula migrating upward and laterally) cannot be executed.

Unilateral shortening causes a head tilt and postural scoliosis.

Weakness: Unilateral reduction in strength leads to postural scoliosis of the cervical spine, with convexity on the weakened side.

The descending part of the trapezius and the levator scapulae are auxiliary respiratory muscles. If the patient uses these muscles, respiratory volume will be reduced. This occurs in patients with upper cervical spinal cord injuries, for example.

1. Palpation of the descending part of the trapezius and the levator scapulae muscles is performed with the patient prone.
   The transverse part of the trapezius and the rhomboid will be easiest to palpate when they are actively performing their primary action (posteromedial movement of the scapula) (see pp. 130 and 131).
2. The patient is prone, with the arms next to the body (**Fig. 69 a**). The patient shrugs the shoulders toward the head. Movement is always tested on both sides.
3. The patient sits on a stool, with the arms hanging down next to the body (**Fig. 69 b**).
4. 5. 6. Starting position is the same as for grade 3 (**Fig. 69 c**). The examiner presses down on the shoulders.

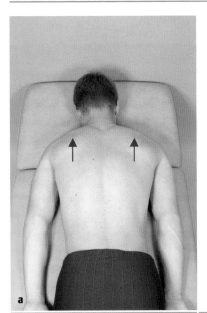

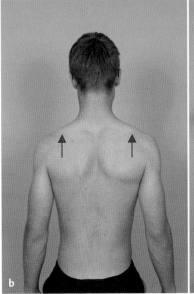

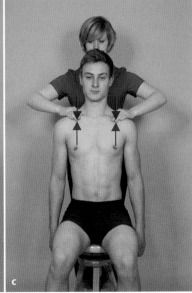

Fig. 69 Functional testing of scapular elevation for grades 2, 3, 4, 5, and 6.

■ Depression of the Scapula (Fig. 70)

	Muscle	Origin	Insertion
1	*Trapezius muscle (ascending part)* Accessory nerve and ramus trapezius (C2–C4)	Spinal processes of T3–T12 vertebrae, supraspinal ligaments	Scapular spine
	Latissimus dorsi muscle Thoracodorsal nerve (C6–C8)	Spinal processes of T7–T12 vertebrae, thoracolumbar fascia, posterior third of the iliac crest	Crest of lesser tubercle
	Pectoralis major muscle Pectoral nerves (C5–T1)	Medial half of clavicle, sternal membrane, cartilage of second to sixth ribs, anterior leaf of rectus sheath	Crest of greater tubercle
2	*Anterior serratus muscle* Long thoracic nerve (C5–C7)	First to ninth ribs	Medial border of scapula
	Pectoralis minor muscle Pectoral nerves (C6–C8)	Third to fifth ribs	Coracoid process
	Subclavius muscle Subclavian nerve (C5–C6)	Cartilage–bone border of first rib	Subclavian groove of clavicle

Clinical Symptoms

Shortening: Isolated shortening of the ascending part of the trapezius muscle is extremely rare. Clinical symptoms of the other muscles involved in scapular depression are described under their primary function.

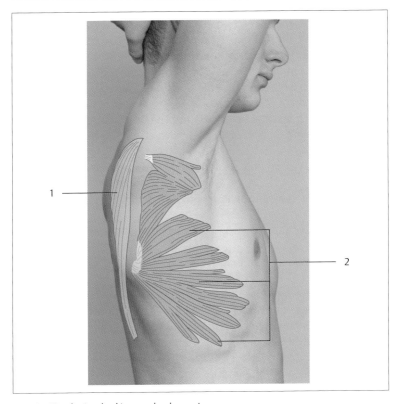

Fig. 70 Muscles involved in scapular depression:
1   Trapezius muscle (ascending part)
2   Anterior serratus muscle

Weakness: Scapular depression is required in order to raise the arm beyond 70°. If these muscles are weakened, the patient will attempt to compensate by extending and lateral bending of the trunk. In addition, the patient will raise his or her shoulder, in order to extend the range of motion.

1̄ Palpation of the ascending part of the trapezius muscle is performed with the patient prone. Contraction can be palpated between the inferior angle of the scapula and the vertebral column.

The subclavian muscle is a weak, thin muscle and can be palpated only in the clavipectoral triangle, since it is covered by the pectoralis major over most of its course.

It is easier to test the innervation of the other muscles involved in this movement when they are actively performing their primary action:

- latissimus dorsi muscle (shoulder extension, see pp. 138 and 139)
- pectoralis major muscle (shoulder adduction, see pp. 146 and 147)
- anterior serratus muscle (scapular abduction, see pp. 126 and 127)
- pectoralis minor muscle (scapular abduction, see pp. 126 and 127).

2̄ The patient is prone, with the arms next to the body (**Fig. 71 a**).
The examiner moves the scapula down and back toward the spine. For this evaluation, only a partial movement is performed.

3̄ Starting position and movement are the same as for grade 2. The full range of motion is achieved.

4̄ 5̄ 6̄ Starting position and movement are the same as for grade 3 (**Fig. 71 b**).
The examiner applies resistance to the inferior angle of the scapula.

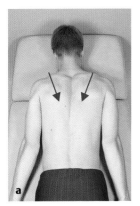 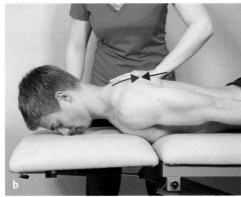

Fig. 71 Testing of scapular depression for grades 2, 3, 4, 5, and 6.

■ Abduction (Protraction) of the Scapula (Fig. 72)

	Muscle	Origin	Insertion
1	*Anterior serratus muscle* Long thoracic nerve (C5–C7)	First to ninth ribs	Medial border of scapula
2	*Pectoralis major muscle* Pectoral nerves (C5–T1)	Medial half of clavicle, sternal membrane, cartilage of second to sixth ribs, anterior leaf of rectus sheath	Crest of greater tubercle
3	*Pectoralis minor muscle* Pectoral nerves (C6–C8)	Third to fifth ribs	Coracoid process

Clinical Symptoms

Shortening: The shoulders are protracted and the thoracic spine has an exaggerated kyphotic curvature.

The antagonists—muscles that adduct the scapula—are in a continuously stretched position, since their insertion and origin are far away from each other, owing to the lateralization of the scapula. They tend to be very weak.

In the shoulder joint, forward flexion, abduction, and external rotation movements are limited.

Weakness: In addition to pulling the scapula forward, the anterior serratus muscle also presses the scapula against the thorax. If this muscle is weak, this movement is incomplete, leading to the clinical symptoms of winged scapula (see pp. 246–249), which is most pronounced when the patient lifts the arm while holding a weight.

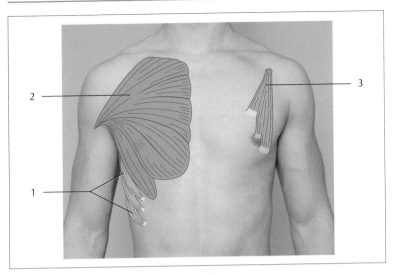

Fig. 72 Muscles involved in abducting the scapula:
1   Anterior serratus muscle
2   Pectoralis major muscle
3   Pectoralis minor muscle

1. The examiner palpates the anterior serratus and pectoralis minor muscles, with the patient seated at the end of the treatment table. The patient's arm on the side to be tested is placed on the treatment table in 90° forward flexion (**Fig. 73 a**).

   Contraction of the anterior serratus muscle can be palpated laterally at the first nine ribs anterior to the scapula.

   The pectoralis minor muscle can be palpated anteriorly and medially, below the coracoid process.

   It is easier to palpate the pectoralis major muscle when it is actively performing its primary function (arm adduction, see pp. 146 and 147).

2. The patient sits at the end of the treatment table. The patient's arm on the side to be tested is placed on the treatment table in 90° forward flexion (**Fig. 73 a**). The examiner stabilizes the opposite shoulder and stabilizes the thorax posteriorly at the lower costal margin on the side to be tested. The examiner can place a cloth between the arm and table to reduce friction. The patient pushes the arm and scapula forward. During the movement, the arm remains in 90° forward flexion.

3. The patient is supine. The shoulder joint is flexed forward to 90° and the elbow is flexed (**Fig. 73 b**). The examiner can stabilize the lower border of the thorax on the side to be tested.

   From this position, the patient pushes the elbow up. The shoulder joint remains in 90° flexion during this movement.

4. 5. 6. Starting position and stabilization are the same as for grade 3. The examiner applies resistance to the elbow (**Fig. 73 c**). The examiner should be aware that the patient will attempt to abduct the arm to gain leverage against the examiner's resistance.

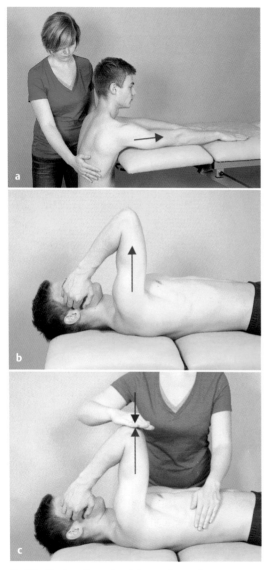

Fig. 73 Testing of scapular abduction for grades 2, 3, 4, 5, and 6.

■ Adduction (Retraction) of the Scapula (Fig. 74)

	Muscle	Origin	Insertion
1	Trapezius muscle		
	Descending part	Superior nuchal line, external occipital protuberance, ligamentum nuchae	Lateral third of clavicle
	Transverse (middle) part	Spinal processes of C7–T3 vertebrae, supraspinal ligaments	Acromial end of clavicle, acromion, scapular spine
	Ascending part	Spinal processes of T3–T12 vertebrae, supraspinal ligaments	Scapular spine
	Accessory nerve and ramus trapezius (C2–C4)		
2	Rhomboid muscles	Spinal processes of C6, C7, and T1–T4 vertebrae	Medial border of scapula
	Dorsal scapular nerve (C4–C5)		
3	Latissimus dorsi muscle	Spinal processes of T7–T12 vertebrae, thoracolumbar fascia, posterior third of iliac crest	Crest of lesser tubercle
	Thoracodorsal nerve (C6–C8)		

Clinical Symptoms

Shortening: Shortening of the muscles that adduct (retract) the scapula is very rare.

Weakness: The shoulders are protracted; in many cases, the kyphotic curvature of the thoracic spine is exaggerated.

When the patient lifts the arms, the medial border of the scapula moves away from the thorax wall because the scapula is not attached to the thorax. These symptoms become more pronounced as the muscles become weaker. This is especially apparent when the patient lifts objects from the ground, and can lead to signs of strain on all structures of the shoulder girdle.

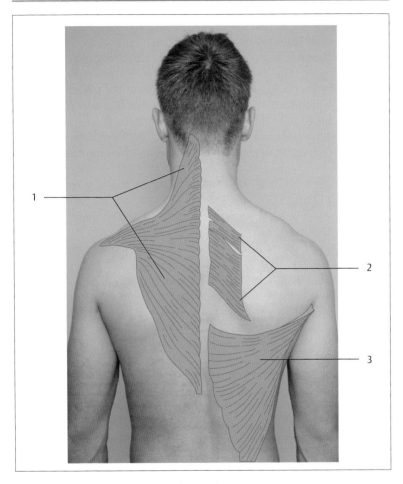

Fig. 74 Muscles involved in adducting the scapula:
1   Trapezius muscle
2   Rhomboid muscles
3   Latissimus dorsi muscle

⬚1 The examiner palpates the muscles that adduct the scapula, with the patient sitting at the end of the treatment table. The patient's arm on the side being tested rests on the treatment table in 90° forward flexion (**Fig. 75a** for grade 2).

The examiner palpates the transverse part of the trapezius muscle and the rhomboid muscles between the medial border of the scapula and the upper thoracic spine.

The following muscles, which participate in this movement, will be easier to palpate when they are actively performing their primary action:

- trapezius muscle, descending part (scapular elevation, see pp. 118 and 119)
- trapezius muscle, ascending part (scapular depression, see pp. 122 and 123)
- latissimus dorsi muscle (shoulder extension, see pp. 138 and 139).

⬚2 The patient sits at the end of the treatment table. The patient's arm on the side being tested rests on the treatment table in 90° forward flexion (**Fig. 75a**). The examiner stabilizes the opposite shoulder and the thorax posteriorly at the lower costal margin on the side being tested. The examiner can place a cloth between the arm and the table to reduce friction.

The patient pulls the scapula back toward the spine. The arm remains in 90° forward flexion during this movement.

⬚3 The patient lies prone at the edge of the treatment table. The patient's arm on the side being tested hangs over the edge of the treatment table in 90° forward flexion (**Fig. 75b**).

The patient pulls the scapula back toward the spine. The arm remains in 90° forward flexion during this movement.

⬚4 ⬚5 ⬚6 Starting position is the same as for grade 3 (**Fig. 75c**).

The examiner applies resistance to the medial border of the scapula.

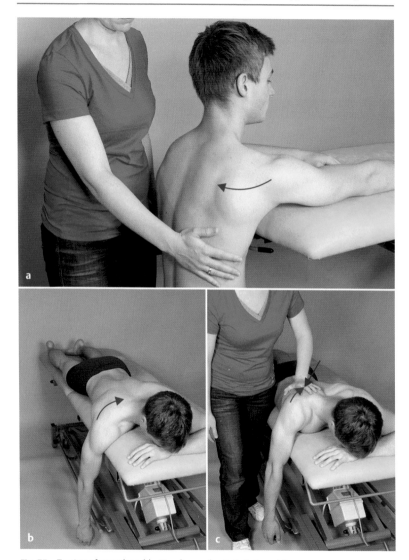

Fig. 75 Testing of scapular adduction for grades 2, 3, 4, 5, and 6.

Shoulder Joint

■ Forward Flexion of the Shoulder Joint (Fig. 76)

	Muscle	Origin	Insertion
1	*Deltoid muscle*		
	Acromial part	Acromion	Deltoid tuberosity
	Axillary nerve (C4–C6)		
	Clavicular part	Lateral third of clavicle	Deltoid tuberosity
	Axillary nerve (C4–C6), pectoral branches (C4–C6)		
2	*Biceps brachii muscle*		
	Long head	Supraglenoid tubercle	Radial tuberosity, antebrachial fascia
	Short head	Coracoid process	Radial tuberosity, antebrachial fascia
	Musculocutaneous nerve (C5–C6)		
3	*Pectoralis major muscle*		
	Clavicular head	Medial third of clavicle	Crest of greater tubercle
	Sternocostal head	Sternal membrane, cartilage of second to sixth ribs	Crest of greater tubercle
	Pectoral nerves (C5–T1)		
	Coracobrachialis muscle	Coracoid process	Medial surface of humerus
	Musculocutaneous nerve (C6–C8)		
	Supraspinatus muscle	Supraspinous fossa	Superior facet of greater tubercle
	Suprascapular nerve (C4–C6)		

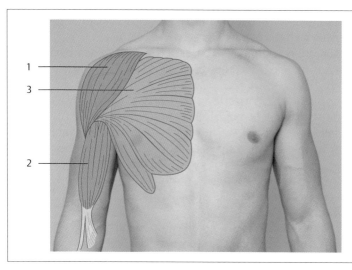

Fig. 76 Muscles involved in forward flexion of the shoulder joint:
1 Deltoid muscle
2 Biceps brachii muscle
3 Pectoralis major muscle

Clinical Symptoms

Shortening: The pectoralis major and biceps brachii muscles are often shortened.

When this is the case, the shoulder will be protracted. In the shoulder joint, forward flexion, abduction, extension, and external rotation movements will be limited. The contracture is often accompanied by weak scapular adductors and external shoulder joint rotators.

Weakness: The patient attempts to compensate for weakening of these muscles by raising the shoulders, bending back the upper body (exaggerating the lordotic curve of the lumbar spine), and increasing lateral bending (convexity on the affected side) of the trunk. By using these compensatory mechanisms, the patient achieves what appears to be a larger range of motion.

If the deltoid and supraspinatus muscles are paretic, subluxation of the humeral head can often be observed, with a characteristic "dent" below the acromion, in addition to flattening of the shoulder profile (see pp. 250 and 251).

[1] The examiner palpates the muscles that participate in flexing the shoulder, with the patient seated.

The supraspinatus muscle is covered by the descending part of the trapezius muscle, which makes it very difficult to palpate its contraction.

The coracobrachialis muscle and the short tendon of the biceps brachii muscle cannot be palpated separately.

The following muscles, which participate in this movement, will be easier to palpate when they are actively performing their primary action, if the examiner is not sure about their innervation:

- biceps brachii muscle (elbow flexion, see pp. 162 and 163)
- pectoralis major muscle (shoulder adduction, see pp. 146 and 147).

Synergy. From around 40° onward, the descending and ascending parts of the trapezius and anterior serratus muscles work in synergy to elevate the shoulder joint. They allow the scapula to rotate about 60°. During the rotation, the inferior angle of the scapula migrates upward and forward.

Unilateral full range of motion requires lateral bending toward the opposite side, with accompanying spinal rotation and extension.

[2] The patient lies on one side. The examiner stabilizes the shoulder on the acromion of the arm being tested, which lies on top (**Fig. 77 a**). For the movement, the patient brings the arm forward on a smooth surface (board), up to around 90°.

[3] The test is performed with the patient seated. The examiner stabilizes the shoulder on the acromion and, if necessary, also stabilizes the patient's upper body (**Fig. 77 b**).

The patient brings the arm forward up to an angle of around 90°.

[4] [5] [6] Starting position and stabilization are the same as for grade 3 (**Fig. 77 c**). The examiner applies resistance to the distal end of the upper arm.

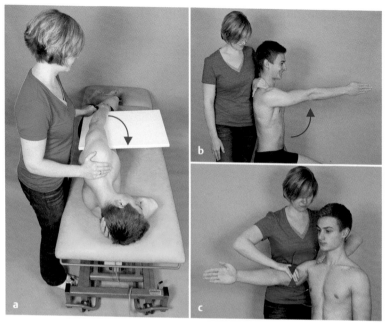

Fig. 77 Testing of forward flexion of the shoulder joint for grades 2, 3, 4, 5, and 6.

■ Extension in the Shoulder Joint (Fig. 78)

	Muscle	Origin	Insertion
1	Teres major muscle	Inferior angle, lateral border of the scapula	Crest of lesser tubercle
	Thoracodorsal nerve (C6–C7)		
2	Latissimus dorsi muscle	Spinal processes of T7–T12 vertebral bodies, thoracodorsal fascia, posterior third of iliac crest	Crest of lesser tubercle
	Thoracodorsal nerve (C6–C8)		
3	Triceps brachii muscle		
	Long head	Infraglenoid tubercle of scapula	Olecranon of ulna
	Radial nerve (C6–C8)		
4	Deltoid muscle		
	Spinal part	Lower border of scapular spine	Deltoid tuberosity
	Acromial part	Acromion of scapula	Deltoid tuberosity
	Axillary nerve (C4–C6)		
	Teres minor muscle	Lateral border of scapula	Inferior facet of greater tubercle
	Axillary nerve (C5–C6)		

Clinical Symptoms

Shortening: Shortening of the teres major and minor, latissimus dorsi, and triceps brachii muscles leads to limited forward flexion.

When the teres major and latissimus dorsi muscles are shortened, external rotation is also limited.

Internal rotation is limited when the teres minor muscle is contracted.

When the patient attempts to lift the arm completely with the elbow flexed, shortening in the triceps brachii becomes particularly apparent.

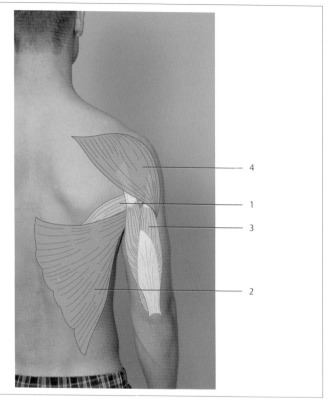

Fig. 78   Muscles involved in shoulder extension:
1   Teres major muscle
2   Latissimus dorsi muscle
3   Triceps brachii muscle
4   Deltoid muscle

All of these contractures lead to disturbances in scapulohumeral rhythm during arm movements and therefore disturb the synergy. This can result in overloading of the other muscles that move or stabilize the shoulder joint.

Weakness: Weakness of muscles that extend the shoulder joint is initially manifested during extreme loading, such as when the patient attempts to support himself or herself on both arms or do chin-ups.

1 The examiner palpates the muscles responsible for shoulder extension, with the patient seated.
   If the innervation of the triceps brachii muscle is unclear, it will be easier to palpate it when it is actively performing its primary action (elbow extension, see pp. 158 and 159).

Synergy. The rhomboid muscles and the transverse part of the trapezius muscle work in synergy during extension of the shoulder joint. They adduct and stabilize the scapula. This function is required to create a basis for the muscles that are acting to perform the movement.

2 The patient lies on the side that is not being tested. The examiner stabilizes the tested shoulder on the acromion (**Fig. 79 a**).
   The patient pulls back the arm on a flat surface (board), to around 45° extension.

3 The patient lies prone, with the arm hanging next to the treatment table (Fig. **79 b**). The examiner stabilizes the side being tested at the acromion.
   The patient brings the arm alongside the thorax, up to an angle of around 45°.
   If the triceps brachii muscle is not strong enough to keep the elbow joint extended during the movement, the patient can also keep the elbow flexed during the test.

4 5 6 Starting position and stabilization are the same as for grade 3 (**Fig. 79 c**).
   The examiner applies resistance to the back of the distal end of the upper arm.

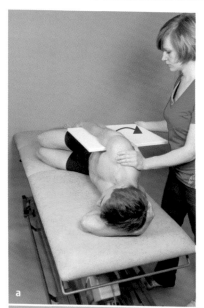

Fig. 79 Testing shoulder joint extension for grades 2, 3, 4, 5, and 6.

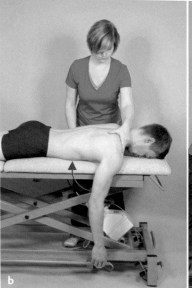

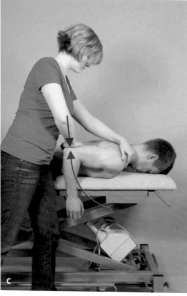

■ Abduction in the Shoulder Joint (Fig. 80)

	Muscle	Origin	Insertion
1	Deltoid muscle		
	Acromial part	Acromion of scapula	Deltoid tuberosity
	Axillary nerve (C4–C6)		
	Spinal part	Lower border of scapular spine	Deltoid tuberosity
	Axillary nerve (C4–C6)		
	Clavicular part	Lateral third of clavicle	Deltoid tuberosity
	Axillary nerve (C4–C6), pectoral branches (C4–C6)		
2	Supraspinatus muscle	Supraspinous fossa	Superior facet of greater tubercle
	Suprascapular nerve (C4–C6)		
	Biceps brachii muscle		
	Long head	Supraglenoid tubercle	Radial tuberosities, antebrachial fascia
	Musculocutaneous nerve (C5–C6)		

Clinical Symptoms

Shortening: Contractures of the deltoid muscle are very rare, while contractures of the long tendon of the biceps brachii muscle are more common.

Weakness: Flattening of the shoulder profile is striking, along with the typical "dent" below the acromion, with subluxation of the humeral head.

The patient attempts to compensate for weakening of these muscles by raising the shoulders and by increasing lateral bending (convexity on the affected side) of the trunk. By using these compensatory mechanisms, the patient achieves what appears to be a larger range of motion (see pp. 250 and 251).

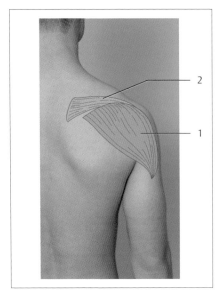

Fig. 80 Muscles involved in shoulder abduction:
1   Deltoid muscle
2   Supraspinatus muscle

1 The examiner palpates the shoulder abductors, with the patient supine.

The supraspinatus muscle is located beneath the descending part of the trapezius muscle and is difficult to palpate.

If the innervation of the biceps brachii muscle is unclear, it will be easier to palpate it when it is actively performing its primary action (elbow flexion, see pp. 162 and 163).

Synergy. Pure abduction in the shoulder joint occurs during the first 90° of movement, up to where the major tubercle meets the superior border of the joint socket. The test is conducted within this range of motion.

However, the scapula already starts participating in this movement (rotation), starting at 30°. From 90° onward, the movement consists of scapula movement and an accompanying movement of the spinal column (lateral bending toward the opposite side). During the scapular movement, the inferior angle migrates forward and upward. The descending and ascending parts of the trapezius and anterior serratus muscles are required for this movement. They also act in synergy during abduction of the shoulder joint.

2 The patient is supine, with the arm being tested resting next to the body on a towel. The examiner stabilizes the shoulder on the acromion (**Fig. 81 a**).

With the wrist in a neutral position, the patient abducts the arm to 90°.

3 The test is performed with the patient seated and the arm hanging next to the body. The examiner stabilizes the shoulders at the acromion (**Fig. 81 b**).

The patient lifts the arm out to the side, to approximately 90° abduction, while maintaining the wrist in a neutral position.

4 5 6 Starting position and stabilization are the same as for grade 3 (**Fig. 81 c**). The examiner applies resistance to the distal end of the upper arm.

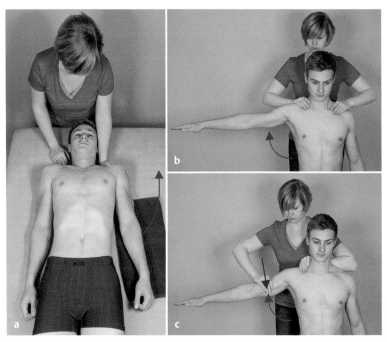

Fig. 81 Testing of shoulder abduction for grades 2, 3, 4, 5, and 6.

■ Adduction in the Shoulder Joint (Fig. 82)

	Muscle	Origin	Insertion
1	*Pectoralis major muscle*	Medial half of clavicle, sternal membrane, cartilage of second to sixth ribs, anterior leaf of rectus sheath	Crest of greater tubercle
	Pectoral nerves (C5–T1)		
2	*Triceps brachii muscle*		
	Long head	Infraglenoid tubercle	Olecranon
	Radial nerve (C6–C8)		
3	*Teres major muscle*	Lateral border of scapula	Crest of lesser tubercle
	Thoracodorsal nerve (C6–C7)		
4	*Latissimus dorsi muscle*	Spinal processes of T7–T12 vertebrae, thoracolumbar fascia, posterior third of iliac crest, tenth to twelfth ribs	Crest of lesser tubercle
	Thoracodorsal nerve (C6–C8)		
	Deltoid muscle		
	Clavicular part	Lateral third of clavicle	Deltoid tuberosity
	Axillary nerve (C4–C6), pectoral branches (C4–C6)		
	Spinal part	Lower border of scapular spine	Deltoid tuberosity
	Axillary nerve (C4–C6)		
	Biceps brachii muscle		
	Short head	Coracoid process	Radial tuberosity, antebrachial fascia
	Musculocutaneous nerve (C5–C6)		

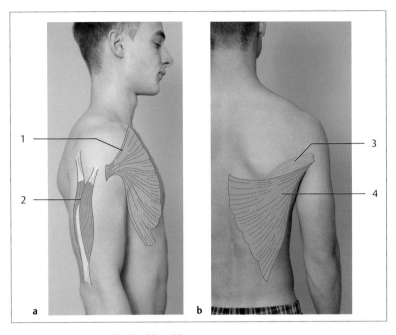

Fig. 82 Muscles involved in shoulder adduction:
1   Pectoralis major muscle
2   Triceps brachii muscle
3   Teres major muscle
4   Latissimus dorsi muscle

Muscle	Origin	Insertion
Coracobrachialis muscle	Coracoid process	Medial surface of humerus
Musculocutaneous nerve (C5–C6)		
Subscapularis muscle	Subscapular fossa	Lesser tubercle of humerus, crest of lesser tubercle
Subscapular nerve (C5–C8)		

Clinical Symptoms

Shortening: The pectoralis major muscle is frequently affected. Contracture leads to a protracted shoulder position.

Symptoms may also include the following:

- exaggerated kyphotic curvature in the thoracic spine, with a more pronounced cervical lordosis as a compensatory measure
- stretched and weakened muscles that adduct and lower the scapula
- weak cervical spine flexors and thoracic spine extensors
- secondary shortening of the pectoralis minor muscle, the short head of the biceps brachii muscle, the coracobrachialis muscle, the descending part of the trapezius muscle, and the cervical spine extensors.

Shortening of the muscles that adduct the shoulder joint, with the above-described accompanying symptoms, limits the shoulder's range of motion in all directions. External rotation, abduction, and forward flexion are particularly affected.

Weakness: Symptoms do not occur unless the muscles are strongly exerted, for instance, when the patient does chin-ups or supports him or herself on the arms.

1 The examiner palpates the muscles that adduct the glenohumeral joint, with the patient seated.
If the innervation is not clear, the following muscles that participate in this movement will be easier to palpate when they are actively performing their primary action:
- biceps brachii muscle (elbow flexion, see pp. 162 and 163)
- coracobrachialis muscle (forward flexion of the shoulder joint, see p. 134)
- clavicular part of the deltoid muscle (forward flexion of the shoulder joint, see pp. 134 and 135)
- spinal part of the deltoid muscle (extension of the shoulder joint, see pp. 138 and 139).

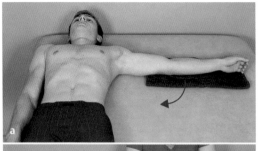

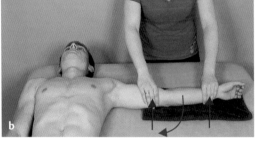

Fig. 83 Testing of shoulder adduction for grades 2, 3, 4, 5, and 6.

Synergy. The synergistic muscles (rhomboid and trapezius muscles) attach the scapula to the thorax, thus forming a stable basis for arm adduction.

2̲ The patient is supine, with the arm abducted to 90°. The patient moves the arm closer to the body (**Fig. 83a**). The examiner places a cloth between the arm and the table, to reduce friction during the movement.

3̲ This movement cannot be tested against gravity. The starting position is therefore the same as for grade 2. Instead of gravity, appropriate resistance is applied by the examiner distally to the inside of the upper arm.

4̲ 5̲ 6̲ Starting position is the same as for grade 2 (**Fig. 83b**). For each test, the examiner applies the required resistance distally to the inside of the upper arm.

■ External Rotation in the Shoulder Joint (Fig. 84)

	Muscle	Origin	Insertion
1	*Infraspinatus muscle*	Infraspinous fossa, scapular spine, infraspinous fascia	Greater tubercle
	Suprascapular nerve (C4–C6)		
2	*Teres minor muscle* Axillary nerve (C5–C6)	Lateral border of scapula	Greater tubercle
3	*Deltoid muscle*		
	Spinal part	Inferior border of scapular spine	Deltoid tuberosity
	Axillary nerve (C4–C6)		

Clinical Symptoms

Shortening: The external rotators of the shoulder are rarely shortened because the shoulder joint at rest sits in approximately 30° internal rotation.

However, they can be shortened after long periods of immobilization, which limits their ability to internally rotate the arm.

Weakness: During shoulder abduction, the infraspinatus and teres minor muscles, along with the subscapularis muscle (internal rotator), jointly center the humeral head in the socket. Depending on the degree of weakness, this function cannot be sufficiently executed when the patient lifts his or her arm. The loss in muscle strength makes itself known when the patient performs tasks requiring stamina and repetitive movements (e.g., washing windows). The patient attempts to compensate for this weakness by increasing the use of the abductors (overloading the supraspinatus muscle), raising the shoulder (overloading the levator scapulae muscle, in the descending part of the trapezius muscle), and increasing lateral bending of the trunk.

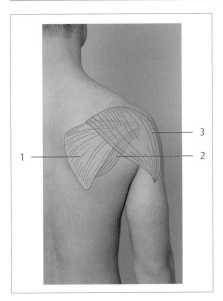

Fig. 84   Muscles involved in externally rotating the shoulder joint:
1   Infraspinatus muscle
2   Teres minor muscle
3   Deltoid muscle

[1] The examiner palpates the shoulder external rotators, with the patient prone. The patient's arm is resting in 90° abduction on the treatment table, with the shoulder externally rotated.

Synergy. External rotation in the glenohumeral joint requires scapular adduction. Muscles working in synergy are the rhomboid, latissimus dorsi, and trapezius muscles. If these muscles are weak, the patient will usually present with winged scapula.

[2] The patient lies prone, with the arm hanging off the treatment table (**Fig. 85 a**). The shoulder joint is flexed 90° and the elbow is flexed 90°. The examiner stabilizes the arm on the side being tested, in a way that stops the patient from raising his or her torso, but still letting the scapula move freely.
The patient maintains the shoulder and elbow in the flexed position and then turns the arm outward.

[3] The patient is prone, with the upper arm next to the treatment table and the shoulder abducted 90° (**Fig. 85 b**). The elbow is flexed 90° and the lower arm hangs over the edge of the treatment table. The examiner stabilizes the torso as described for evaluation of grade 2 muscle strength.
The patient turns his or her arm upward, while maintaining the flexed position.

[4] [5] [6] Starting position and stabilization are the same as for grade 3 (**Fig. 85 c**). The examiner applies resistance to the back of the forearm, near the wrist.

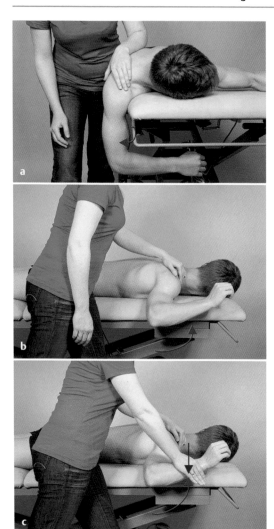

Fig. 85   Testing of external rotation in the shoulder joint for grades 2, 3, 4, 5, and 6.

■ Internal Rotation in the Shoulder Joint (Fig. 86)

	Muscle	Origin	Insertion
1	*Subscapularis muscle*	Subscapular fossa	Lesser tubercle of humerus, crest of lesser tubercle
	Subscapular nerve (C5–C8)		
2	*Pectoralis major muscle*	Medial half of clavicle, sternal membrane, cartilage of second to sixth ribs, anterior leaf of rectus sheath	Crest of greater tubercle
	Pectoral nerves (C5–T1)		
	Biceps brachii muscle		
	Long head	Supraglenoid tubercle	Radial tuberosity, antebrachial fascia
	Musculocutaneous nerve (C5–C6)		
	Deltoid muscle		
	Clavicular part	Lateral third of clavicle	Deltoid tuberosity
	Pectoral branches (C4–C6), axillary nerve (C4–C6)		
	Teres major muscle	Lateral border of scapula	Crest of lesser tubercle
	Thoracodorsal nerve (C6–C7)		
3	*Latissimus dorsi muscle*	Spinal processes of T7–T12 vertebrae, thoracolumbar fascia, posterior third of iliac crest, tenth to twelfth ribs	Crest of lesser tubercle
	Thoracodorsal nerve (C6–C8)		

Clinical Symptoms

Shortening: There may be limitations in external rotation and forward flexion, as well as abduction.

A secondary symptom is shortening of the synergists and anterior serratus and pectoralis minor muscles.

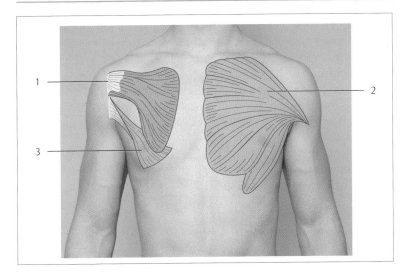

Fig. 86 Muscles involved in internal rotation of the shoulder joint:
1   Subscapularis muscle
2   Pectoralis major muscle
3   Latissimus dorsi muscle

Owing to scapular lateralization, these contractures cause constant hyperextension. This, in turn, weakens the antagonists, i.e., the muscles that adduct and depress the scapula.

The external rotators of the scapula are also affected, owing to overextension and weakness.

Thoracic spine extension may be reduced and cervical spine lordosis increased. If the contracture persists, the cervical spine extensors shorten and the cervical spine flexors become weaker.

These complex changes can limit shoulder movements in every direction.

Weakness: Weakening of the shoulder internal rotators is rare and manifests itself only when they are placed under extreme loads.

This may be due to the fact that the arms mainly move in flexion and internal rotation during daily activities.

[1] Since the subscapularis muscle is located below the shoulder blade and covered by the spinal part of the deltoid muscle near its insertion, it is very difficult to palpate. Palpation is performed with the patient supine.

If the examiner is not sure about innervation, contraction of all the other muscles involved in internally rotating the shoulder joint will be easier to test when they are actively performing their primary action:

- biceps brachii muscle (elbow flexion, see pp. 162–165)
- clavicular part of the deltoid muscle (forward flexion of the shoulder joint, see pp. 134–137)
- teres major muscle (extension of the shoulder joint, see pp. 138–141)
- latissimus dorsi muscle (extension of the shoulder joint, see pp. 138–141).

Synergy. Internal rotation in the shoulder joint requires scapular abduction. The anterior serratus and pectoralis minor muscles are therefore required synergists.

[2] The patient lies prone, with the arm hanging next to the treatment table in 90° flexion and maximum external rotation (**Fig. 87 a**). The elbow is flexed at 90°. If the patient is unable to hold this position actively, the examiner must support the forearm in this position.

The examiner stabilizes the scapula in a way that stops the patient raising his or her torso, but still lets the scapula move freely.

The patient maintains the shoulder and elbow in the flexed position and then turns the arm inward.

[3] The patient is prone, with the upper arm resting on the treatment table and the shoulder joint abducted to 90° (**Fig. 87 b**). The lower arm hangs over the side of the table and the elbow is flexed 90°. The examiner stabilizes the scapula in a way that stops the patient raising his or her torso, but still lets the scapula move freely. During internal rotation, the patient maintains the flexed position in the shoulder and elbow joints.

[4] [5] [6] Starting position and stabilization are the same as for grade 3 (**Fig. 87 c**). The examiner applies the required resistance distally to the inside of the forearm.

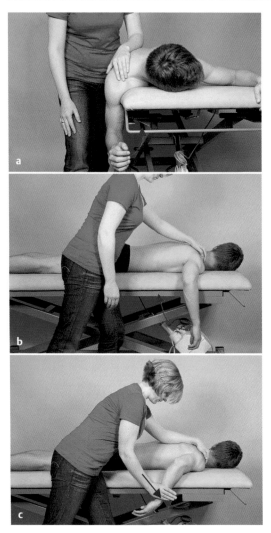

Fig. 87 Testing of internal rotation in the shoulder joint for grades 2, 3, 4, 5, and 6.

Elbow

■ Extension in the Elbow (Fig. 88)

	Muscle	Origin	Insertion
1	*Triceps brachii muscle*		
	Medial head	Distally from radial groove of posterior surface of humerus, medial and lateral intermuscular septum	Olecranon, posterior wall of capsule
	Lateral head	Laterally and proximally from radial groove of posterior surface of humerus	Olecranon, posterior wall of capsule
	Long head	Infraglenoid tubercle of scapula	Olecranon, posterior wall of capsule
	Radial nerve (C6–C8)		
2	*Anconeus muscle*	Posterior surface of lateral epicondyle, lateral collateral ligament	Proximal quarter of posterior ulna
	Radial nerve (C7–C8)		

Clinical Symptoms

Shortening: The long head of the triceps brachii muscle is a bi-articular muscle. In addition to extending the elbow joint, it extends and adducts the shoulder joint.

Therefore, shortening is accompanied by limited range of motion, not only when the patient flexes the elbow, but also when he or she elevates and abducts the shoulder joint.

Weakness: Weakened elbow joint extensors manifest themselves only when they are subjected to high levels of loading, such as when performing push-ups.

If these muscles do not function at all, the patient will use a trick to compensate for it: he or she will rotate the shoulder joint externally, supinate the forearm, and in so doing, achieve passive extension in the elbow.

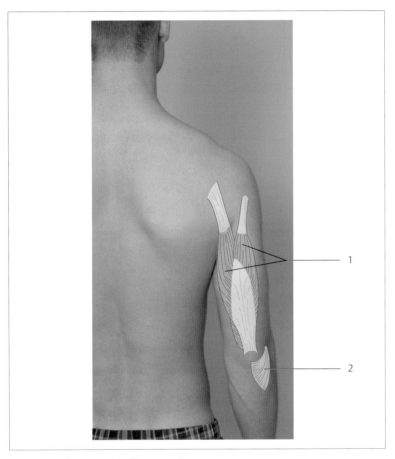

Fig. 88 Muscles involved in elbow extension:
1   Triceps brachii muscle
2   Anconeus muscle

[1] The examiner palpates the elbow extensors, with the patient seated. The patient's shoulder is abducted 90° and the arm rests on the treatment table. Elbow joint flexion must be adjusted individually to the most favorable angle for contraction. The examiner stabilizes the upper arm (**Fig. 89 a** for grade 2).

[2] The patient is seated, with the shoulder abducted 90° and the forearm resting on the treatment table (**Fig. 89 a**). The elbow joint is flexed as much as possible and the forearm placed in a neutral position. The examiner can place a cloth under the forearm to reduce friction during the movement. The examiner stabilizes the upper arm.

The patient extends his or her elbow, while keeping the forearm in a neutral position.

[3] The patient lies prone, with the forearm hanging next to the treatment table. The examiner stabilizes the upper arm (**Fig. 89 b**).

The patient extends his or her elbow, while keeping the forearm in a neutral position.

[4][5][6] Starting position and stabilization are the same as for grade 3 (**Fig. 89 c**). The examiner applies resistance to the ulnar side of the forearm.

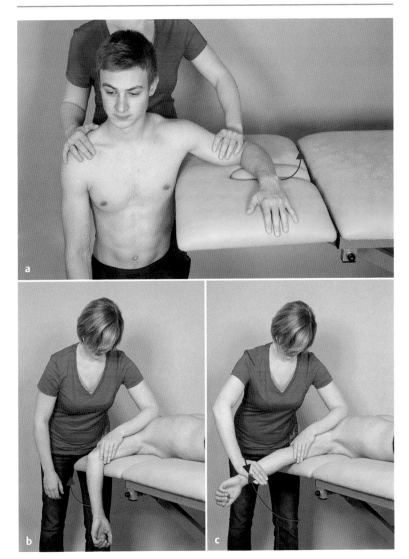

Fig. 89   Testing of elbow extension for grades 2, 3, 4, 5, and 6.

■ Flexion in the Elbow (Fig. 90)

	Muscle	Origin	Insertion
1	*Biceps brachii muscle*		
	Long head	Supraglenoid tubercle	Radial tuberosity, antebrachial fascia
	Short head	Coracoid process	Radial tuberosity, antebrachial fascia
	Musculocutaneous nerve (C5–C6)		
2	*Brachialis muscle*	Anterior surface of humerus, intermuscular septa	Tuberosity of ulna, joint capsule
	Musculocutaneous nerve (C5–C6)		
3	*Brachioradialis muscle*	Medial supra-epicondylar ridge, lateral intermuscular septum	Radial styloid process
	Radial nerve (C5–C6)		
	Extensor carpi radialis longus muscle	Lateral supra-epicondylar ridge, lateral intermuscular septum	Base of second metacarpal
	Radial nerve (C5–C7)		
4	*Pronator teres muscle (humeral head)*	Medial epicondyle of humerus, medial intermuscular septum	Lateral surface of radius
	Median nerve (C6–C7)		
	Flexor carpi radialis muscle	Medial epicondyle of humerus, surface of forearm fascia	Palmar surface of base of second metacarpal
	Median nerve (C6–C8)		
	Extensor carpi radialis brevis muscle	Lateral epicondyle of humerus, annular ligament of radius, radial collateral ligament	Base of second metacarpal
	Radial nerve (C7)		

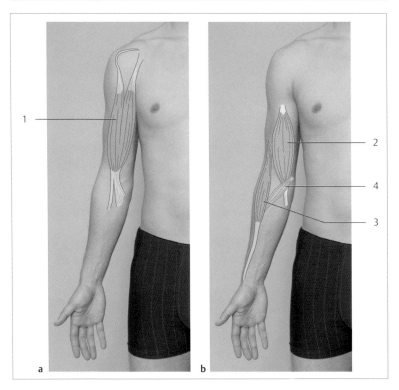

Fig. 90 Muscles involved in elbow joint flexion:
1   Biceps brachii muscle
2   Brachialis muscle
3   Brachioradialis muscle
4   Pronator teres muscle

Clinical Symptoms

Shortening: The biceps brachii muscle is a bi-articular muscle. It is involved in flexion of the elbow joint, as well as in forward flexion and internal rotation in the shoulder joint.

Shortening of this muscle manifests itself as limited extension of the elbow joint, and also limited shoulder extension and external rotation.

Shortening of the participating forearm muscles is described in the section on wrist extension and flexion.

Weakness: Weakness of the elbow joint flexors is apparent especially when the patient lifts heavy objects.

The patient is unable to compensate for complete functional loss. However, he or she will attempt to minimize the influence of gravity by means of shoulder abduction and lateral bending (convexity on the affected side) of the trunk, in order to facilitate the flexion.

1. The examiner palpates the elbow joint flexors, with the patient seated. The arm is abducted 90° and rests on the treatment table (**Fig. 91 a** for grade 2).
   The elbow joint is extended. The patient may need to flex the joint slightly, so the examiner can palpate a contraction in the biceps brachii muscle.
   If the innervation is not clear, the following muscles that participate in this movement will be easier to palpate when they are actively performing their primary action:
   - extensor carpi radialis longus and brevis muscles (wrist extension, see pp. 174–177)
   - pronator teres muscle (distal and proximal radioulnar joint pronation, see pp. 170–173)
   - flexor carpi radialis muscle (wrist flexion, see pp. 178–181).

2. The patient is seated, with the arm abducted 90° and resting on the treatment table (**Fig. 91 a**). The elbow joint is extended and the forearm is in a neutral position. The examiner stabilizes the upper arm and the shoulder.
   The examiner can place a cloth under the forearm to prevent friction during testing.
   The patient flexes his or her elbow through the full range of motion, while maintaining the forearm in a neutral position.

3. The patient is seated, with the arm hanging next to the body (**Fig. 91 b**). The examiner presses and stabilizes the upper arm against the patient's body.
   The patient lifts the forearm, while keeping it in a neutral position.

4. 5. 6. Starting position is the same as for evaluation of grade 3 muscle strength (**Fig. 91 c**). The examiner stabilizes the patient's upper arm with his or her body.
   The examiner applies resistance to the radial side of the forearm, proximal to the wrist.

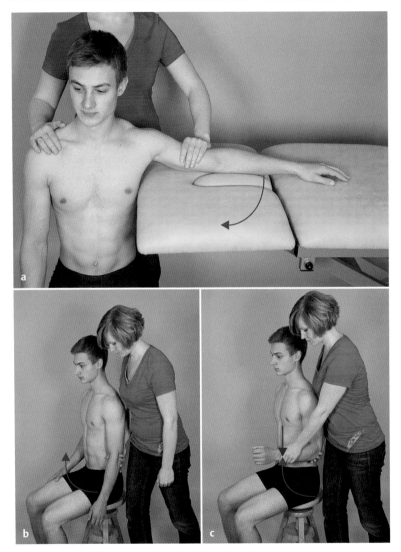

Fig. 91   Testing of elbow flexion for grades 2, 3, 4, 5, and 6.

■ Supination of the Distal and Proximal Radioulnar Joint (Fig. 92)

	Muscle	Origin	Insertion
	Supinator muscle	Supinator crest of ulna, lateral epicondyle of humerus, lateral collateral ligament, annular ligament of radius	Radius
	Radial nerve (C5–C6)		
1	*Biceps brachii muscle*		
	Long head	Supraglenoid tubercle	Radial tuberosity, antebrachial fascia
	Short head	Coracoid process	Radial tuberosity, antebrachial fascia
	Musculocutaneous nerve (C5–C6)		
	Abductor pollicis longus muscle	Posterior surface of ulna, interosseous membrane, posterior surface of radius	Base of first metacarpal
	Radial nerve (C7–C8)		
	Extensor pollicis longus muscle	Posterior surface of ulna, interosseous membrane	Base of distal thumb phalanx
	Radial nerve (C7–C8)		
	Brachioradialis muscle	Lateral supra-epicondylar ridge, lateral intermuscular septum	Radial styloid process
	Radial nerve (C5–C6)		

Clinical Symptoms

Shortening: The biceps brachii and brachioradialis muscles supinate the forearm and flex the elbow joint. If these muscles are shortened, the range of motion during forearm pronation and elbow extension will be limited. The patient compensates for the limited pronation movement by increasing internal rotation and abduction of the shoulder. This brings about lateral bending of the trunk, with convexity toward the affected side.

Weakness: Weakness of the forearm supinators manifests itself during various everyday movements, such as tightening a screw, turning a doorknob, or closing a faucet.

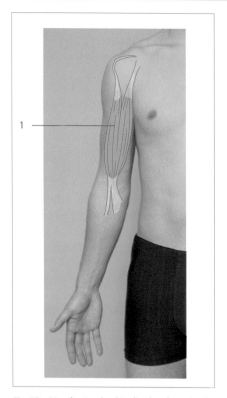

Fig. 92   Muscles involved in distal and proximal radioulnar joint supination:
1   Biceps brachii muscle

1 The examiner palpates the forearm supinators, with the patient's forearm resting on the treatment table in slight pronation.

The supinator muscle cannot be palpated, owing to the extensors covering it.

The brachioradialis muscle is only involved in forearm supination movement from the pronated position up to the neutral position of the forearm.

The strength of the biceps brachii muscle during supination increases with greater elbow flexion. It is greatest at 90° flexion and then diminishes again with further flexion.

The following muscles that participate in this movement will be easier to palpate when they are actively performing their primary action, if the examiner is not sure about their innervation:

- biceps brachii muscle (elbow flexion, see pp. 162 and 163)
- abductor pollicis longus muscle (thumb carpometacarpal joint abduction, see pp. 202 and 203)
- extensor pollicis longus muscle (thumb carpometacarpal joint extension, see pp. 190 and 191)
- brachioradialis muscle (elbow flexion, see pp. 162 and 163).

2 The patient's upper arm rests on the treatment table and the elbow joint is flexed 90° (**Fig. 93 a**). The examiner stabilizes the distal end of the upper arm.

The patient executes the movement over a full range of motion from pronation to supination.

3 Since the muscle cannot be tested against gravity, the starting position and stabilization are the same as for grade 2 (**Fig. 93 b**).

Instead of gravity, appropriate resistance is applied by the examiner at the distal end of the forearm.

4 5 6 Starting position and stabilization are the same as for grade 2. The examiner applies resistance to the distal end of the forearm.

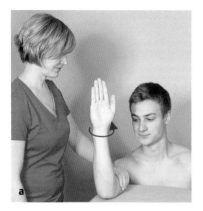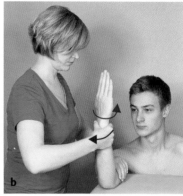

Fig. 93   Testing of distal and proximal radioulnar joint supination for grades 2, 3, 4, 5, and 6.

■ Pronation of the Distal and Proximal Radioulnar Joint (Fig. 94)

	Muscle	Origin	Insertion
1	*Pronator quadratus muscle*	Distal quarter of palmar surface of ulna	Distal quarter of palmar surface of radius
	Median nerve (C8–T1)		
2	*Pronator teres muscle*		
	Humeral head	Medial epicondyle of humerus, medial intermuscular septum	Lateral surface of radius
	Ulnar head	Coronoid process of ulna	Lateral surface of radius
	Median nerve (C6–C7)		
3	*Flexor carpi radialis muscle*	Medial epicondyle of humerus, surface of antebrachial fascia	Palmar surface of base of second metacarpal
	Median nerve (C6–C8)		
	Extensor carpi radialis longus muscle	Lateral supra-epicondylar ridge, lateral intermuscular septum	Palmar surface of base of second metacarpal
	Radial nerve (C5–C7)		
4	*Brachioradialis muscle*	Lateral supra-epicondylar ridge, lateral intermuscular septum	Radial styloid process
	Radial nerve (C5–C6)		

Clinical Symptoms

Shortening: In addition to limited supination, shortening of the muscles that produce pronation also limits the range of motion in elbow extension because all muscles cross the elbow joint and produce flexion, except the pronator quadratus muscle.

In everyday life, this makes it difficult to perform functions such as turning a key or tightening a screw. The patient compensates for this limited range of motion by increasing shoulder external rotation and adduction and through lateral bending of the trunk.

Weakness: When performing certain everyday functions, the patient lacks the strength to turn the faucet or loosen a screw, for example.

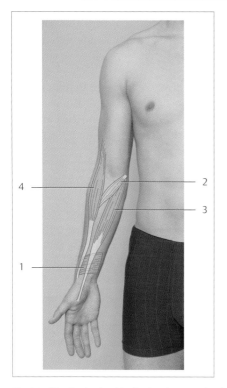

Fig. 94 Muscles involved in distal and proximal radioulnar joint pronation:
1   Pronator quadratus muscle
2   Pronator teres muscle
3   Flexor carpi radialis muscle
4   Brachioradialis muscle

[1] The examiner palpates the forearm pronators, with the patient's forearm resting on the treatment table in slight supination.

The pronator quadratus muscle is difficult to palpate because it is covered by the finger and wrist flexors.

The brachioradialis muscle is only involved in the pronation movement from the supination position up to the neutral position of the forearm. It will be easier to test the following muscles for contraction when they are actively performing their primary action, if the examiner is not sure about their innervation:

- flexor carpi radialis muscle (wrist flexion, see pp. 178 and 179)
- extensor carpi radialis longus muscle (wrist extension, see pp. 174 and 175)
- brachioradialis muscle (elbow flexion, see pp. 162 and 163)
- palmaris longus muscle (wrist flexion, see pp. 178 and 179).

[2] The patient's upper arm rests on the treatment table and the elbow joint is flexed 90° (**Fig. 95 a**). The examiner stabilizes the distal end of the upper arm.

The patient executes the movement over a full range of motion from supination to pronation.

[3] Since the muscle cannot be tested against gravity, the starting position and stabilization are the same as for grade 2 (**Fig. 95 b**).

Instead of gravity, appropriate resistance is applied by the examiner to the distal end of the forearm.

[4][5][6] Starting position and stabilization are the same as for grade 2. The examiner applies resistance to the distal end of the forearm.

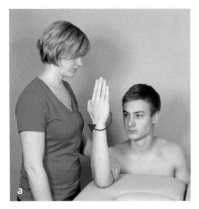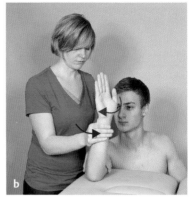

Fig. 95   Testing of distal and proximal radioulnar joint pronation for grades 2, 3, 4, 5, and 6.

Wrist

■ Extension of the Wrist (Fig. 96)

	Muscle	Origin	Insertion
1	*Extensor digitorum muscle*	Lateral epicondyle of humerus, lateral collateral ligament, annular ligament of radius, antebrachial fascia	Bases of proximal phalanges, posterior aponeuroses of second to fifth fingers
	Radial nerve (C6–C8)		
2	*Extensor carpi radialis longus muscle*	Lateral supra-epicondylar ridge, lateral intermuscular septum	Base of second metacarpal
	Radial nerve (C5–C7)		
3	*Extensor carpi radialis brevis muscle*	Common head of lateral epicondyle of humerus, lateral collateral ligament, annular ligament of radius	Base of third metacarpal
	Radial nerve (C7)		
4	*Extensor indicis muscle*	Posterior surface of ulna, interosseous membrane	Posterior aponeurosis of index finger
	Radial nerve (C8–T1)		
5	*Extensor pollicis longus muscle*	Posterior surface of ulna, interosseous membrane	Base of distal phalanx of thumb
	Radial nerve (C7–C8)		
6	*Extensor digiti minimi muscle*	Common head of lateral epicondyle of humerus	Posterior aponeurosis of fifth finger
	Radial nerve (C6–C8)		

Clinical Symptoms

Shortening: Wrist flexion and flexion in all fingers is limited.

Shortening of the wrist extensors is evident if the wrist and fingers flex when the elbow is extended. When an individual performs everyday ac-

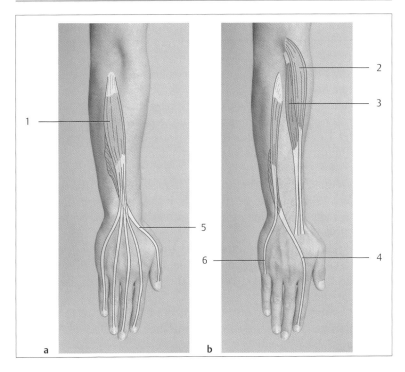

Fig. 96   Muscles involved in wrist extension:
1   Extensor digitorum muscle
2   Extensor carpi radialis longus muscle
3   Extensor carpi radialis brevis muscle
4   Extensor indicis muscle
5   Extensor pollicis longus muscle
6   Extensor digiti minimi muscle

tivities, shortening is not noticeable. However, if it is combined with persistent overloading of the wrist extensors, it can cause lateral epicondylitis (tennis elbow).

Weakness: Patients cannot maintain wrist extension with a pronated forearm while lifting heavy objects. The wrist tilts toward the volar side. If the patient frequently lifts objects in this position, overloading symptoms may occur at the origin tendons of the finger and wrist extensors (lateral epicondylitis).

1️⃣ The examiner palpates the wrist extensors, with the patient's forearm resting on the treatment table in pronation. The examiner supports the forearm distally. Depending on the patient's ability to contract the muscle, the examiner holds the wrist in neutral or in slight extension.

It is easier to palpate the extensor digitorum, extensor indicis, and extensor digiti minimi muscles with the patient's fingers extended and it is easier to palpate the extensor pollicis longus muscle with the thumb interphalangeal joint extended.

2️⃣ The patient's forearm rests on the treatment table in a neutral position (**Fig. 97 a**), with the examiner stabilizing it near the wrist. The fingers will flex as the wrist extends. If the finger flexors are overly tight, the wrist's range of motion into extension will be negatively affected.

3️⃣ The patient's forearm rests on the treatment table in pronation, with the hand hanging over the edge (**Fig. 97 b**). The examiner stabilizes the forearm near the wrist. The patient extends the wrist by flexing the fingers.

4️⃣5️⃣6️⃣ Starting position and stabilization are the same as for grade 3 (**Fig. 97 c**). The examiner applies resistance to the back of the hand.

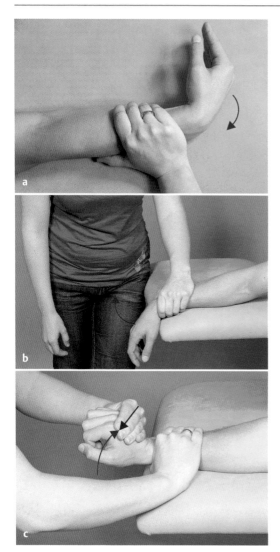

Fig. 97 Testing of wrist extension for grades 2, 3, 4, 5, and 6.

■ Flexion of the Wrist (Fig. 98)

	Muscle	Origin	Insertion
1	*Flexor digitorum superficialis muscle* Median nerve (C7–T1)	Medial epicondyle of humerus, coronoid process of ulna, radius	Center of medial phalanges of second to fifth fingers
2	*Flexor digitorum profundus muscle* Median nerve and ulnar nerve (C6–T1)	Palmar surface of ulna, interosseous membrane	Bases of distal phalanges of second to fifth fingers
3	*Flexor carpi ulnaris muscle* Ulnar nerve (C7–C8)	Medial epicondyle of humerus, olecranon, upper two-thirds of posterior border of ulna	Pisiform bone
4	*Flexor pollicis longus muscle* Median nerve (C7–C8)	Anterior surface of radius, interosseous membrane	Distal thumb phalanx
5	*Flexor carpi radialis muscle* Median nerve (C6–C8)	Medial epicondyle of humerus, antebrachial fascia	Palmar surface of base of second metacarpal
	Abductor pollicis longus muscle Radial nerve (C8–T1)	Posterior surface of ulna, interosseous membrane, posterior surface of radius	Base of first metacarpal

Clinical Symptoms

Shortening: Limited range of motion during extension of the wrist and all fingers.

Shortening will be more evident if the patient extends the fingers and wrist at the same time as extending the elbow joint.

Clinically, and when performing everyday activities, shortening is unremarkable. However, if it is combined with persistent overloading of the wrist flexors, it can cause medial epicondylitis (golfer's elbow).

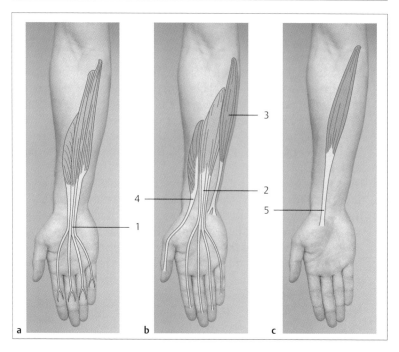

Fig. 98   Muscles involved in wrist flexion:
1   Flexor digitorum superficialis muscle
2   Flexor digitorum profundus muscle
3   Flexor carpi ulnaris muscle
4   Flexor pollicis longus muscle
5   Flexor carpi radialis muscle

Weakness: When the patient lifts heavy objects with the forearm supinated, he or she is unable to sufficiently stabilize the wrist in flexion. The wrist tilts dorsally. If there are repeated loads in this joint position, overloading symptoms may occur at the origin tendons of the finger and wrist flexors (medial epicondylitis).

[1] The examiner palpates the wrist flexors, with the patient's forearm resting on the treatment table in supination. The examiner stabilizes the forearm in this position.

It is easier to test the contractibility of the flexor digitorum superficialis muscle and the flexor digitorum profundus muscle in combination with finger flexion. Likewise, it is easier to test the contractibility of the flexor pollicis longus muscle together with flexion in the metacarpophalangeal joint, and of the abductor pollicis longus muscle together with abduction in the thumb carpometacarpal joint.

[2] The patient's forearm rests on the treatment table in a neutral position (**Fig. 99 a**), with the examiner stabilizing it near the wrist.

[3] The patient's forearm rests on the treatment table in supination, with the hand hanging over the edge (**Fig. 99 b**).

The examiner stabilizes the forearm near the wrist.

[4] [5] [6] Starting position and stabilization are the same as for grade 3 (**Fig. 99 c**). The examiner applies resistance to the palm of the patient's hand.

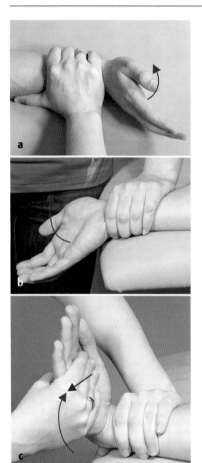

Fig. 99   Testing of wrist flexion for grades 2, 3, 4, 5, and 6.

■ Radial Deviation (Abduction) of the Wrist (Fig. 100)

	Muscle	Origin	Insertion
1	Extensor carpi radialis longus muscle Radial nerve (C5–C7)	Lateral supra-epicondylar ridge, lateral intermuscular septum	Base of first metacarpal
2	Abductor pollicis longus muscle Radial nerve (C8–T1)	Posterior surface of ulna, interosseous membrane, posterior surface of radius	Base of first metacarpal
	Extensor pollicis longus muscle Radial nerve (C7–C8)	Posterior surface of ulna, interosseous membrane	Base of distal thumb phalanx
3	Flexor carpi radialis muscle Median nerve (C6–C8)	Medial epicondyle of humerus, forearm fascia	Palmar surface of base of second metacarpal
	Flexor pollicis longus muscle Median nerve (C6–C8)	Anterior surface of radius, interosseous membrane	Base of distal thumb phalanx
	Extensor pollicis brevis muscle Radial nerve (C7–T1)	Ulna, interosseous membrane, posterior surface of radius	Base of proximal thumb phalanx

Clinical Symptoms

Shortening: In addition to limited ulnar deviation, shortening can also limit wrist extension and flexion.

Weakness: Weakness during radial deviation in the wrist may occur in combination with weakness in wrist extension or flexion.

It clearly manifests itself when the patient lifts objects with the forearm in a neutral position.

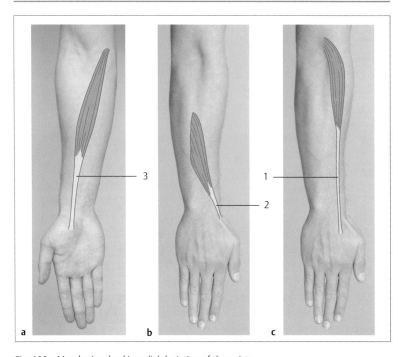

Fig. 100 Muscles involved in radial deviation of the wrist:
1   Extensor carpi radialis longus muscle
2   Abductor pollicis longus muscle
3   Flexor carpi radialis muscle

1. It is easier to test all of the muscles involved in radial deviation of the wrist for contractibility when they are actively performing their primary action:
   - extensor carpi radialis longus muscle (wrist extension, see pp. 174 and 175)
   - abductor pollicis longus muscle (abduction in the thumb carpometacarpal joint, see pp. 202 and 203)
   - extensor pollicis longus muscle (extension in the thumb metacarpophalangeal joint, see pp. 190 and 191)
   - flexor carpi radialis muscle (wrist flexion, see pp. 178 and 179)
   - flexor pollicis longus muscle (flexion in the thumb metacarpophalangeal joint, see pp. 192 and 193).

2. The patient's forearm rests on the treatment table, in pronation (**Fig. 101 a**). The examiner stabilizes the forearm near the wrist.
   The patient executes the movement from ulnar deviation to radial deviation. The examiner can place a cloth under the hand to reduce friction during the movement.

3. The patient's forearm is placed in a neutral position, with the hand hanging over the edge of the treatment table (**Fig. 101 b**). The examiner stabilizes the forearm near the wrist.

4. 5. 6. Starting position and stabilization are the same as for grade 3 (**Fig. 101 c**).
   The examiner applies resistance to the first metacarpal.

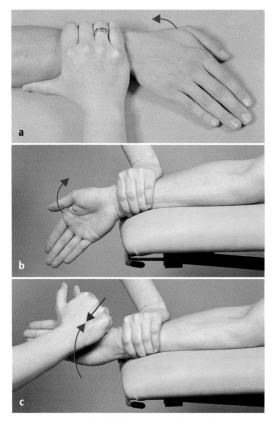

Fig. 101   Testing of radial deviation in the wrist for grades 2, 3, 4, 5, and 6.

■ Ulnar Deviation (Adduction) of the Wrist (Fig. 102)

	Muscle	Origin	Insertion
1	*Extensor carpi ulnaris muscle* Radial nerve (C7–C8)	Lateral epicondyle of humerus, posterior surface of ulna	Base of fifth metacarpal
2	*Flexor carpi ulnaris muscle* Ulnar nerve (C7–C8)	Medial epicondyle of humerus, olecranon, upper two-thirds of posterior border of ulna	Pisiform bone
	Extensor digitorum muscle Radial nerve (C6–C8)	Lateral epicondyle of humerus, lateral collateral ligament, annular ligament of radius, antebrachial fascia	Bases of proximal phalanges, posterior aponeuroses of second to fifth fingers
	Extensor digiti minimi muscle Radial nerve (C6–C8)	Lateral epicondyle of humerus	Posterior aponeurosis of fifth finger

Clinical Symptoms

Shortening: In addition to limiting radial deviation, shortening will also affect wrist extension and flexion.

Weakness: Weakness during ulnar deviation in the wrist always occurs in combination with weakness during wrist extension or flexion.

Reduced strength related to ulnar deviation has little functional impact.

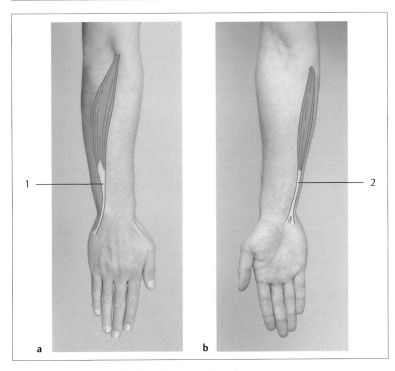

a   b

Fig. 102 Muscles involved in ulnar deviation of the wrist:
1   Extensor carpi ulnaris muscle
2   Flexor carpi ulnaris muscle

[1] Except for the extensor carpi ulnaris muscle, it will be easier to test the contractibility of all the other muscles involved in ulnar deviation when they are performing their primary function:

- flexor carpi radialis muscle (wrist flexion, see pp. 178 and 179)
- extensor digitorum muscle (finger extension, see pp. 228 and 229)
- extensor digiti minimi muscle (extension of the 5th finger, see pp. 228 and 229).

[2] The patient's forearm rests on the treatment table, in pronation (**Fig. 103 a**), with the examiner stabilizing it near the wrist.

The patient executes the movement from radial deviation to ulnar deviation. The examiner can place a cloth under the forearm to reduce friction during the movement.

[3] The patient is seated, with the arm hanging next to the body. The examiner stabilizes the forearm in pronation near the wrist at the patient's body (**Fig. 103 b**).

[4][5][6] Starting position and stabilization are the same as for grade 3 (**Fig. 103 c**).

The examiner applies resistance to the fifth metacarpal.

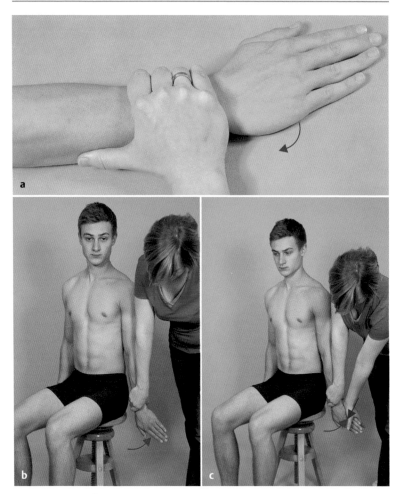

Fig. 103 Testing of ulnar deviation in the wrist for grades 2, 3, 4, 5, and 6.

Thumb Joints

■ Extension in the Interphalangeal Joint of the Thumb (Fig. 104)

	Muscle	Origin	Insertion
1	*Extensor pollicis longus muscle* Radial nerve (C7–C8)	Posterior surface of ulna, interosseous membrane	Base of distal thumb phalanx

Clinical Symptoms

Shortening: Flexion in the metacarpophalangeal and interphalangeal joints of the thumb, as well as opposition, is limited.

Weakness: The patient cannot fully reposition the thumb and is unable to sufficiently open the hand to grasp larger objects. The patient's interphalangeal joint of the thumb is flexed.

[1] The examiner palpates the muscle, with the patient's forearm and hand resting on the treatment table. The examiner stabilizes the metacarpophalangeal joint of the thumb.

[2] The patient's forearm and hand rest on the treatment table. The examiner stabilizes the interphalangeal joint of the thumb (**Fig. 105**). The patient can perform up to half the extension range of motion of the interphalangeal joint of the thumb.

[3] Starting position and stabilization are the same as for evaluation of grade 2 muscle strength.
The patient is able to perform the full range of motion.

[4] [5] [6] Starting position and stabilization are the same as for grade 2. The examiner applies resistance to the dorsal aspect of the distal phalanx of the thumb.

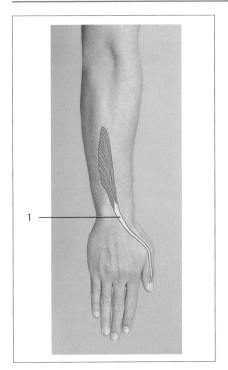

Fig. 104 Muscles involved in extending the interphalangeal joint of the thumb:
1   Extensor pollicis longus muscle

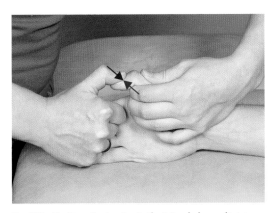

Fig. 105 Testing of extension in the interphalangeal joint of the thumb for grades 2, 3, 4, 5, and 6.

■ Flexion in the Interphalangeal Joint of the Thumb (Fig. 106)

	Muscle	Origin	Insertion
1	*Flexor pollicis longus muscle*	Anterior surface of radius, interosseous membrane	Base of distal thumb phalanx
	Median nerve (C6–C8)		

Clinical Symptoms

Shortening: Shortening of the flexor pollicis longus muscle limits extension in the distal phalanx of the thumb, as well as limiting range of motion when repositioning the thumb.

Weakness: The pincer grasp, a highly significant function, is altered. If there is weakness, the patient will extend the interphalangeal joint of the thumb to grasp items and will increase thumb adduction.

⬜ The examiner palpates the muscle, with the patient's forearm resting on the treatment table in supination. The examiner stabilizes the metacarpophalangeal joint of the thumb in extension.

2️⃣ Starting position and stabilization are the same as for evaluation of grade 1 muscle strength.
The patient can perform up to half the flexion range of motion of the interphalangeal joint of the thumb.

3️⃣ Starting position and stabilization are the same as for grade 2.
The patient is able to perform the full range of motion.

4️⃣5️⃣6️⃣ Starting position and stabilization are the same as for grade 2 (**Fig. 107**). The examiner applies resistance to the dorsal aspect of the distal thumb phalanx.

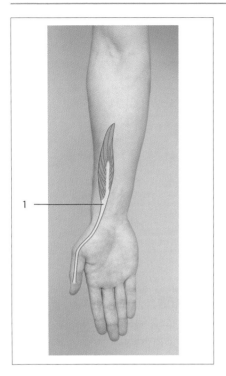

Fig. 106 Muscles involved in flexing the interphalangeal joint of the thumb:
1   Flexor pollicis longus muscle

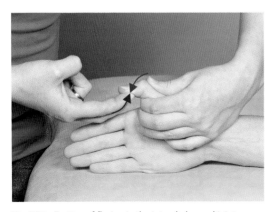

Fig. 107 Testing of flexion in the interphalangeal joint of the thumb for grades 2, 3, 4, 5, and 6.

■ Extension in the Metacarpophalangeal Joint of the Thumb (Fig. 108)

	Muscle	Origin	Insertion
1	*Extensor pollicis longus muscle*	Posterior surface of ulna, interosseous membrane	Base of distal thumb phalanx
	Radial nerve, deep root (C7–C8)		
2	*Extensor pollicis brevis muscle*	Posterior surface of ulna, interosseous membrane, posterior surface of radius	Base of proximal thumb phalanx
	Radial nerve, deep root (C7–C8)		

Clinical Symptoms

Shortening: Flexion in the metacarpophalangeal and interphalangeal joints of the thumb, as well as opposition, is limited.

Weakness: The strength of thumb reposition is reduced. The patient is unable to sufficiently open his or her hand to grasp larger objects.

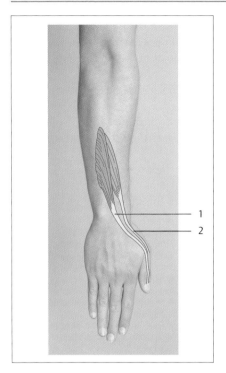

Fig. 108 Muscles that extend the metacarpophalangeal joint of the thumb:
1   Extensor pollicis longus muscle
2   Extensor pollicis brevis muscle

1. The examiner palpates the muscle, with the patient's forearm and hand resting on the treatment table in a neutral position. The examiner stabilizes the carpometacarpal joint of the thumb (**Fig. 109** for grade 2).

   It is easier to palpate the extensor pollicis longus muscle with the thumb interphalangeal joint extended.

2. The patient's forearm and hand rest on the treatment table in a neutral position. The examiner stabilizes the carpometacarpal joint of the thumb (**Fig. 109 a**).

   The patient can perform up to half the extension range of motion for the thumb metacarpophalangeal joint.

3. Starting position and stabilization are the same as for evaluation of grade 2 muscle strength.

   The patient performs the full range of motion.

4. 5. 6. Starting position and stabilization are the same as for grade 2 (**Fig. 109 b**).

   The examiner applies resistance to the dorsal aspect of the proximal thumb phalanx.

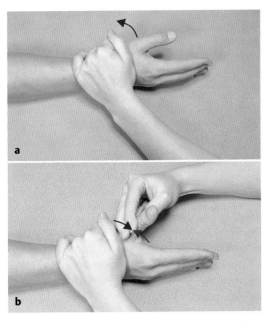

Fig. 109   Testing of extension in the proximal phalanx of the thumb for grades 2, 3, 4, 5, and 6.

■ Flexion in the Metacarpophalangeal Joint of the Thumb (Fig. 110)

	Muscle	Origin	Insertion
1	*Flexor pollicis longus muscle*	Anterior surface of radius, interosseous membrane	Base of distal thumb phalanx
	Anterior interosseus branch of the median nerve (C6–C8)		
2	*Flexor pollicis brevis muscle*		
	Superficial head	Flexor retinaculum	Radial sesamoid bone of thumb metacarpophalangeal joint
	Median nerve (C8–T1)		
	Deep head	Trapezoid bone, trapezium bone, capitate bone	Radial sesamoid bone of thumb metacarpophalangeal joint
	Ulnar nerve (C8–T1)		

Clinical Symptoms

Shortening: Extension in the metacarpophalangeal and interphalangeal joints of the thumb, as well as reposition, is limited.

Weakness: The strength of opposition is reduced. When the patient holds onto an object, the carpometacarpal joint of the thumb will be adducted.

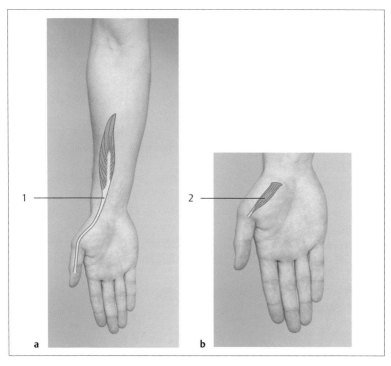

a   b

Fig. 110   Muscles involved in flexing the metacarpophalangeal joint of the thumb:
1   Flexor pollicis longus muscle
2   Flexor pollicis brevis muscle

1 The examiner palpates the muscle, with the patient's supinated forearm resting on the treatment table. The examiner stabilizes the carpometacarpal joint of the thumb (**Fig. 111 a** for grade 2).

The deep head of the flexor pollicis brevis muscle is covered by other muscles and cannot be palpated.

It is easier to palpate the flexor pollicis longus muscle if the thumb interphalangeal joint is also flexed.

2 The patient's forearm rests on the treatment table in supination. The examiner stabilizes the carpometacarpal joint of the thumb (**Fig. 111 a**).

The patient can perform up to half the flexion range of motion in the thumb metacarpophalangeal joint.

3 Starting position and stabilization are the same as for evaluation of grade 2 muscle strength.

The patient is able to perform the full range of motion.

4 5 6 Starting position and stabilization are the same as for grade 2 (**Fig. 111 b**).

The examiner applies resistance to the volar aspect of the proximal thumb phalanx.

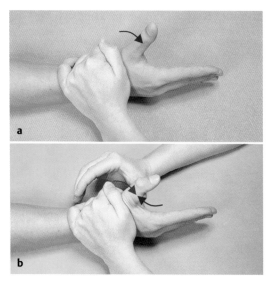

Fig. 111 Testing of flexion in the metacarpophalangeal joint of the thumb for grades 2, 3, 4, 5, and 6.

■ Abduction in the Carpometacarpal Joint of the Thumb (Fig. 112)

	Muscle	Origin	Insertion
1	*Abductor pollicis longus muscle* Radial nerve (C7–C8)	Posterior surface of ulna, interosseous membrane, posterior surface of radius	Base of first metacarpal
2	*Abductor pollicis brevis muscle* Median nerve (C8–T1)	Scaphoid bone, flexor retinaculum	Radial sesamoid bone of proximal thumb phalanx
	Extensor pollicis brevis muscle Radial nerve (C7–T1)	Ulna, interosseous membrane, posterior surface of radius	Base of proximal thumb phalanx
	Opponens pollicis muscle Median nerve (C6–C7)	Tubercle of trapezium bone, flexor retinaculum	Radial border of first metacarpal
	Flexor pollicis longus muscle Median nerve (C6–C8)	Anterior surface of radius, interosseous membrane	Base of distal thumb phalanx

> ### Clinical Symptoms
>
> **Shortening:** Shortening of these muscles is rare.
>
> **Weakness:** If the muscle is weakened, the thumb cannot be sufficiently abducted. Opposition and reposition movements of the thumb are limited.
>
> In terms of function, this reduced strength is described as the positive bottle sign: when the patient grasps a bottle or a glass, the distance between the thumb and index finger is reduced, and the web does not touch the object. The ball of the thumb is atrophied.

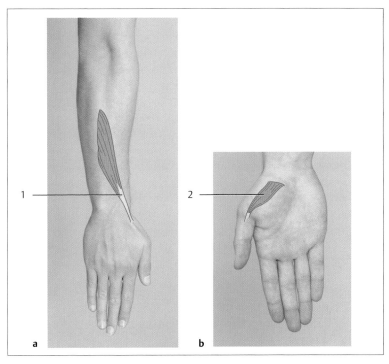

a   b

Fig. 112   Muscles involved in abduction of the thumb carpometacarpal joint of the thumb:
1   Abductor pollicis longus muscle
2   Abductor pollicis brevis muscle

1️⃣ The examiner palpates the muscles, with the patient's forearm and wrist resting on the treatment table in a neutral position. The examiner stabilizes the wrist in this position (**Fig. 113** for grade 2).

The following muscles will be easier to palpate when they are actively performing their primary action:

- extensor pollicis brevis muscle (extension in the metacarpophalangeal joint of the thumb, see pp. 194 and 195)
- opponens pollicis muscle (flexion in the carpometacarpal joint of the thumb, see pp. 214 and 215)
- flexor pollicis longus muscle (flexion in the interphalangeal joint of the thumb, see pp. 192 and 193).

2️⃣ The examiner palpates the muscles, with the patient's forearm and wrist resting on the treatment table in a neutral position. The examiner stabilizes the wrist (**Fig. 113 a**).

The patient can perform up to half the range of motion for thumb abduction.

3️⃣ Starting position and stabilization are the same as for evaluation of grade 2 muscle strength.

The patient is able to perform the full range of motion.

4️⃣5️⃣6️⃣ Starting position and stabilization are the same as for grade 2 (**Fig. 113 b**).

The examiner applies resistance to the radial aspect of the proximal phalanx of the thumb.

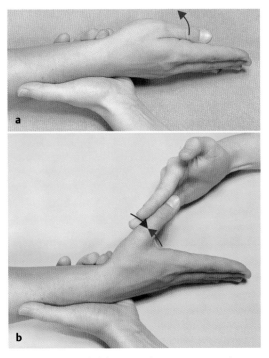

Fig. 113   Testing of abduction in the carpometacarpal joint of the thumb for grades 2, 3, 4, 5, and 6.

■ Adduction in the Carpometacarpal Joint of the Thumb (Fig. 114)

	Muscle	Origin	Insertion
1	Adductor pollicis muscle		
	Transverse head	Third metacarpal	Ulnar sesamoid bone of thumb metacarpophalangeal joint
	Oblique head	Trapezoid bone, capitate bone	Ulnar sesamoid bone of thumb metacarpophalangeal joint
	Ulnar nerve (C8–T1)		
2	Flexor pollicis brevis muscle		
	Superficial head	Flexor retinaculum	Radial sesamoid bone of thumb metacarpophalangeal joint
	Deep head	Trapezium bone, trapezoid bone, capitate bone	Radial sesamoid bone of thumb metacarpophalangeal joint
	Ulnar nerve (C8–T1)		
3	Opponens pollicis muscle	Tubercle of trapezium bone, flexor retinaculum	Radial border of first metacarpal
	Median nerve (C6–C7)		

Clinical Symptoms

Shortening: Limitations in abduction can be expected.

Weakness: Weakness is clearly manifested by atrophy between the first and second metacarpals, especially if there is paresis of the ulnar nerve and the interosseus muscles are also affected.

An easy way to test for weakness is to have the patient hold a sheet of paper using the pincer grasp. When the examiner pulls on the sheet of paper, the patient is unable to maintain the pincer grasp, owing to the weak adductors. The patient attempts to compensate for the weakness by using the flexors more strongly. This causes the thumb interphalangeal joint to become more flexed (positive Froment sign).

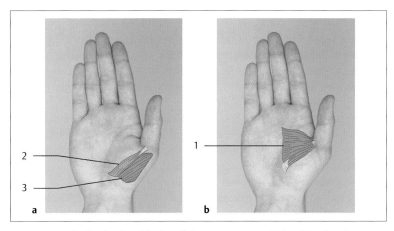

Fig. 114 Muscles involved in adduction of the carpometacarpal joint of the thumb:
1   Adductor pollicis muscle
2   Flexor pollicis brevis muscle
3   Opponens pollicis muscle

1. The examiner palpates the muscles, with the patient's forearm and hand resting on the treatment table in a neutral position. The examiner stabilizes the wrist in extension.

   The deep heads of the flexor pollicis brevis and adductor pollicis muscles are covered by other muscles and therefore very difficult to palpate.

   The superficial head of the flexor pollicis brevis muscle is easier to palpate if the patient flexes the thumb metacarpophalangeal joint. The oppenens pollicis muscle is easier to palpate if the patient flexes the thumb carpometacarpal joint.

2. The patient's forearm and hand rest on the treatment table in a neutral position. The examiner stabilizes the wrist (**Fig. 115a**).

   The patient adducts the thumb from the abduction position up to half the range of motion.

3. Starting position and stabilization are the same as for evaluation of grade 2 muscle strength.

   The patient performs the full range of motion.

4. 5. 6. Starting position and stabilization are the same as for grade 2 (**Fig. 115b**).

   The examiner applies resistance to the ulnar side of the proximal phalanx of the thumb.

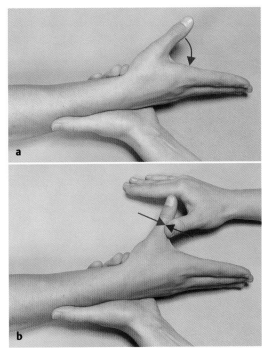

Fig. 115   Testing of adduction in the carpometacarpal joint of the thumb for grades 2, 3, 4, 5, and 6.

■ Extension in the Carpometacarpal Joint of the Thumb (Fig. 116)

	Muscle	Origin	Insertion
1	*Extensor pollicis longus muscle* Radial nerve (C7–C8)	Posterior surface of ulna, interosseous membrane	Base of distal thumb phalanx
2	*Extensor pollicis brevis muscle* Radial nerve (C7–T1)	Ulna, interosseous membrane, posterior surface of radius	Base of proximal thumb phalanx
3	*Abductor pollicis longus muscle* Radial nerve (C7–C8)	Posterior surface of ulna, interosseous membrane, posterior surface of radius	Base of first metacarpal

Clinical symptoms

Shortening: Flexion in the carpometacarpal, metacarpophalangeal, and interphalangeal joints of the thumb is limited, especially when these movements are performed together.

Ulnar deviation in the wrist may also be limited.

Weakness: The strength of the thumb's reposition movement is reduced. The patient is unable to sufficiently open his or her hand to grasp larger objects.

This clinical picture is evident in patients with paresis of the radial nerve (see p. 255).

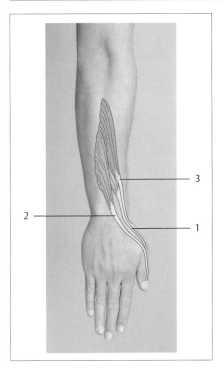

Fig. 116 Muscles involved in extension of the carpometacarpal joint of the thumb:
1   Extensor pollicis longus muscle
2   Extensor pollicis brevis muscle
3   Abductor pollicis longus muscle

1. The examiner palpates the muscle, with the patient's forearm and hand resting on the treatment table in a neutral position. The examiner stabilizes the wrist (**Fig. 117** for grade 2).

   The patient performs the movement in the sagittal plane with the carpometacarpal joint of the thumb slightly abducted. The patient extends the thumb toward the radial side of the wrist.

2. The patient's forearm and hand rest on the treatment table in a neutral position. The examiner stabilizes the wrist in this position (**Fig. 117 a**).

   The movement is described in the test for grade 1 and is performed up to half the range of motion.

3. Starting position and stabilization are the same as for grade 2 evaluation of muscle strength.

   The movement is executed fully.

4. 5. 6. Starting position and stabilization are the same as for grade 2 (**Fig. 117 b**).

   The examiner applies resistance to the dorsal aspect of the first metacarpal.

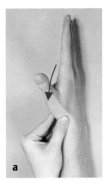
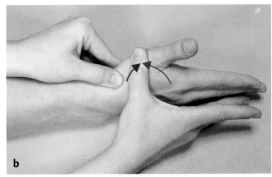

Fig. 117 Testing extension in the carpometacarpal joint of the thumb for grades 2, 3, 4, 5, and 6.

■ Flexion in the Carpometacarpal Joint of the Thumb (Fig. 118)

	Muscle	Origin	Insertion
1	*Flexor pollicis longus muscle*	Anterior surface of radius, interosseous membrane	Base of distal thumb phalanx
	Median nerve (C6–C8)		
2	*Flexor pollicis brevis muscle*		
	Superficial head	Flexor retinaculum of trapezium bone	Radial sesamoid bone of thumb metacarpophalangeal joint
	Median nerve (C8–T1)		
	Deep head	Trapezoid bone, capitate bone	Radial sesamoid bone of the thumb metacarpophalangeal joint
	Ulnar nerve (C8–T1)		
3	*Abductor pollicis brevis muscle*	Scaphoid bone, flexor retinaculum	Radial sesamoid bone of proximal thumb phalanx
	Median nerve (C8–T1)		
4	*Opponens pollicis muscle*	Tubercle of trapezium bone, flexor retinaculum	Radial border of first metacarpal
	Median nerve (C6–C7)		

Clinical Symptoms

Shortening: Extension in the carpometacarpal, metacarpophalangeal, and interphalangeal joints of the thumb is limited.

Depending on the degree of shortening, the patient is unable to sufficiently reposition the thumb. The distance between the thumb and the other fingers diminishes. The patient is unable to grasp larger objects.

Weakness: The strength of the thumb's opposition movement is reduced. When the patient lifts heavier objects, he or she will attempt to compensate for the weakness by increased flexing of the metacarpophalangeal and interphalangeal joints of the thumb.

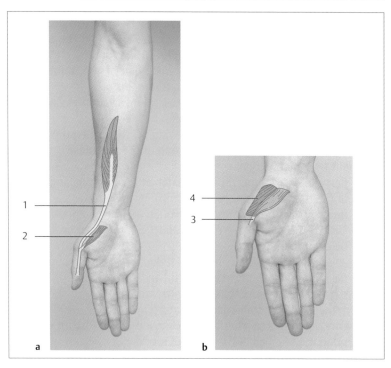

Fig. 118   Muscles involved in flexion of the carpometacarpal joint of the thumb:
1   Flexor pollicis longus muscle
2   Flexor pollicis brevis muscle
3   Abductor pollicis brevis muscle
4   Opponens pollicis muscle

If the flexors are also absent or weakened, the patient will compensate for the absent function by extending the wrist. This passively flexes the metacarpophalangeal and interphalangeal joints of the thumb.

Furthermore, the patient is unable to hold small objects using the pincer grasp and will attempt to compensate for the weakness by adducting the thumb carpometacarpal joint.

This clinical picture is evident in patients with paresis of the median nerve (see pp. 257 and 258).

☐1 The examiner palpates the involved muscles, with the patient's forearm resting on the treatment table in supination. The examiner stabilizes the wrist in this position (**Fig. 119** for grade 2).

The patient flexes the carpometacarpal joint of the thumb in the sagittal plane, with this joint slightly abducted.

It is difficult to differentiate the muscles involved in flexion in the carpometacarpal joint of the thumb.

It will be easier to palpate the following muscles when they are actively performing their primary action, if the examiner is not sure about their innervation:

- flexor pollicis longus muscle (flexion in the interphalangeal joint of the thumb, see pp. 192 and 193)
- flexor pollicis brevis muscle (flexion in the metacarpophalangeal joint of the thumb, see pp. 198 and 199); the deep head cannot be palpated
- abductor pollicis brevis muscle (abduction in the carpometacarpal joint of the thumb, see pp. 202 and 203).

☐2 The patient's forearm rests on the treatment table in supination, with the examiner stabilizing the wrist (**Fig. 119 a**).

The movement is performed as described in the test for grade 1, through the first half of the range of motion.

☐3 Starting position and stabilization are the same as for evaluation of grade 2 muscle strength.

The movement is executed through the full range of motion.

☐4 ☐5 ☐6 Starting position and stabilization are the same as for grade 2 (**Fig. 119 b**).

The examiner applies resistance to the volar aspect of the first metacarpal.

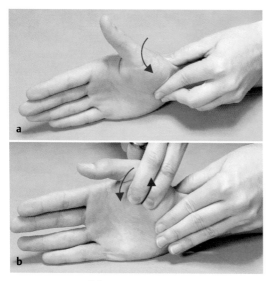

Fig. 119 Testing of flexion in the carpometacarpal joint of the thumb for grades 2, 3, 4, 5, and 6.

Thumb opposition is a combined movement sequence, since the movement requires several joints and a synergy of different functions. For this reason, it cannot be tested directly through manual muscle testing. To make a statement about strength, the test results of all functions involved in opposition must be taken together:

- abduction in the carpometacarpal joint of the thumb—this is a spreading movement of the first metacarpal in the frontal plane
- flexion in the carpometacarpal joint of the thumb—the movement is performed in the abduction position. The patient brings the first metacarpal up to the sagittal plane, which is formed by the second metacarpal
- flexion in the metacarpophalangeal joint of the thumb
- flexion in the interphalangeal joint of the thumb.

A rough functional test for thumb opposition can be performed by having the patient hold an object such as a piece of paper between the thumb and the other fingers.

If there is paresis of the median nerve, the opposition movement will be weakened or absent. Atrophy of the thenar eminence muscles will be evident (see pp. 257 and 258).

Like thumb opposition, *thumb reposition* is a bi-articular movement. It is the result of the synergy of various functions and cannot be tested directly through manual muscle testing. Only evaluation of the functions involved in the movement provides differentiated information about the movement sequence:

- abduction in the carpometacarpal joint of the thumb—this is a spreading movement of the first metacarpal in the frontal plane
- extension in the carpometacarpal joint of the thumb—the movement is performed in the abduction position; the patient extends the thumb toward the radial side
- extension in the metacarpophalangeal joint of the thumb
- extension in the interphalangeal joint of the thumb.

If there is paresis of the radial nerve, thumb reposition will be weakened or completely absent (see p. 255).

Finger Joints

■ Spreading of the Fingers (Fig. 120)

	Muscle	Origin	Insertion
1	*Dorsal interossei muscles*	Aspects of the five metacarpals that face each other	Bases of proximal phalanges, posterior aponeuroses of second to fifth fingers
	Ulnar nerve (C8–T1)		
2	*Abductor digiti minimi muscle*	Pisiform bone, pisohamate ligament, flexor retinaculum	Ulnar border of base of proximal phalanx of fifth metacarpal, extensor aponeurosis of fifth finger
	Ulnar nerve (C8–T1)		
	Extensor digitorum muscle	Lateral epicondyle of humerus, lateral collateral ligament, annular ligament of radius, antebrachial fascia	Bases of proximal phalanges, posterior aponeuroses of second to fifth fingers
	Radial nerve (C6–C8)		

Clinical Symptoms

Shortening: If the dorsal interossei muscles are shortened, the metacarpophalangeal joints of the fingers cannot be extended when the proximal and distal interphalangeal joints are flexed simultaneously. In most cases, the interossei palmares and lumbricals are shortened at the same time.

Weakness: Clear atrophy is visible between the metacarpal bones and at the base of the small finger.

If the dorsal interossei muscles are weakened, the fingers will be in a claw position. This claw position is brought about by overactivity of the extensor digitorum muscles in the metacarpophalangeal joints. They are hyperextended, while the proximal and distal interphalangeal joints are flexed to compensate, owing to the tension of the overextended flexors in the metacarpophalangeal joints.

If the extensor digitorum is weakened, strength will be clearly reduced in all finger joints during extension and during wrist extension.

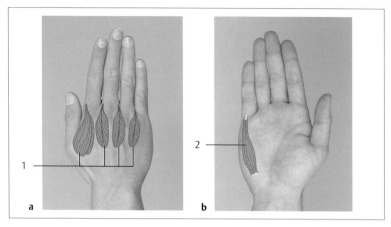

Fig. 120   Muscles involved in spreading the fingers:
1   Dorsal interossei muscles
2   Abductor digiti minimi muscle

⒈ The examiner palpates the muscles, with the patient's forearm resting on the treatment table in pronation. The examiner stabilizes the wrist (**Fig. 121** for grade 2).

⒉ The patient's forearm rests on the treatment table in pronation. The examiner stabilizes the wrist (**Fig. 121 a**).

The patient achieves up to half the range of motion for spreading the fingers.

⒊ Starting position and stabilization are the same as for evaluation of grade 2 muscle strength.

The patient achieves the full range of motion for spreading the fingers.

⒋ ⒌ ⒍ Starting position and stabilization are the same as for grade 2 (**Fig. 121 b**).

For the second finger, the examiner applies resistance to its radial side; for the third finger, to its radial and ulnar side; and for the fourth and fifth finger, to their ulnar side.

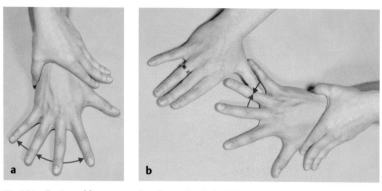

Fig. 121   Testing of finger spreading for grades 2, 3, 4, 5, and 6.

■ Closing of the Fingers (Fig. 122)

	Muscle	Origin	Insertion
1	*Interossei palmares muscles*	Second, fourth, and fifth metacarpal	Bases of the second, third, and fourth proximal phalanges and corresponding dorsal aponeuroses
	Ulnar nerve (C8–T1)		

Clinical Symptoms

Shortening: If the muscles are shortened, the metacarpophalangeal joints cannot be extended when the proximal and distal interphalangeal joints are flexed at the same time. In most cases, the dorsal interossei and lumbricals are shortened at the same time.

Weakness: Strength is reduced during flexion of the metacarpophalangeal joints. A claw position of the fingers is often observed. The metacarpophalangeal joints are hyperextended and the proximal and distal interphalangeal joints are flexed.

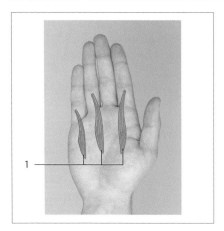

Fig. 122   Muscles involved in closing the fingers:
1   Interossei palmares muscles

[1] The patient's forearm rests on the treatment table, in supination. The examiner stabilizes the wrist (**Fig. 123** for grade 2).

The interossei palmares muscles cannot be palpated. Grade 1 is assigned if there is visible twitching.

[2] The patient's forearm rests on the treatment table, in supination. The fingers are spread and the examiner stabilizes the wrist (**Fig. 123 a**).

The patient partially brings the fingers back together.

[3] Starting position and stabilization are the same as for evaluation of grade 2 muscle strength.

The patient closes the fingers completely.

[4][5][6] Starting position and stabilization are the same as for grade 2 (**Fig. 123 b**).

For the second finger, the examiner applies resistance to its ulnar side, and for the fourth and fifth fingers to their radial side.

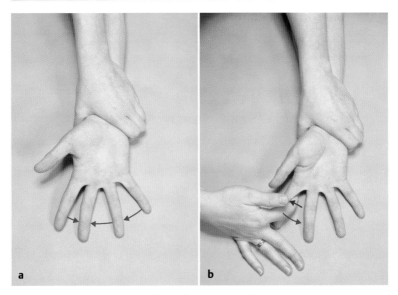

Fig. 123   Testing of finger closing for grades 2, 3, 4, 5, and 6.

■ Extension in the Metacarpophalangeal Joints (Fig. 124)

	Muscle	Origin	Insertion
1	*Extensor digitorum muscle*	Lateral epicondyle of humerus, lateral collateral ligament, annular ligament of radius, antebrachial fascia	Dorsal aponeurosis of second to fifth fingers
	Radial nerve (C6–C8)		
2	*Extensor indicis muscle*	Posterior surface of ulna, interosseous membrane	Dorsal aponeurosis of second finger
	Radial nerve (C6–C8)		
3	*Extensor digiti minimi muscle*	Lateral epicondyle of humerus	Dorsal aponeurosis of fifth finger
	Radial nerve (C6–C8)		

Clinical Symptoms

Shortening: Flexion is limited in all finger joints. Shortening becomes evident when wrist flexion and elbow extension are added. Persistent shortening with simultaneous overloading of these muscles can irritate the origin tendons at the lateral epicondyle.

Weakness: Weakness of the involved muscles, especially the extensor digitorum muscle, leads to weakness in metacarpophalangeal joint extension and reduced strength in wrist extension.

If strength is reduced to an even greater extent, the patient will be unable to actively open his or her hand. In order to grasp objects, the patient will flex the wrist, so that the hand opens passively.

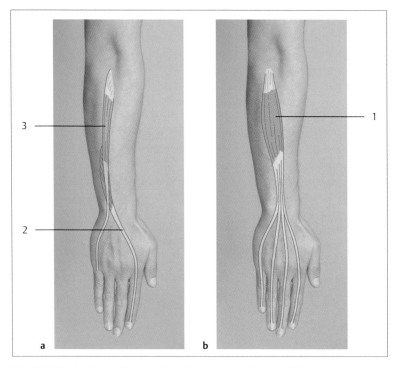

Fig. 124   Muscles involved in extension in the metacarpophalangeal joints:
1   Extensor digitorum muscle
2   Extensor indicis muscle
3   Extensor digiti minimi muscle

1. The examiner palpates the muscles, with the patient's forearm resting on the treatment table in pronation. The examiner holds the hand and stabilizes the wrist in a neutral position. The metacarpophalangeal joints are slightly flexed.

2. The patient's forearm rests on the treatment table, in a neutral position. The examiner stabilizes the wrist (**Fig. 125 a**).

   Depending on the extensibility in the finger flexors, extension of the metacarpophalangeal joints can be performed with the proximal and distal interphalangeal joints either flexed or extended. The movement is executed fully.

3. The patient's forearm rests pronated on the table and the fingers hang over the edge of the treatment table. The examiner stabilizes the wrist (**Fig. 125 b**).

   The metacarpophalangeal joints are fully extended.

4. 5. 6. Starting position and stabilization are the same as for grade 3 (**Fig. 125 c**).

   The examiner applies resistance to the dorsal side of the proximal phalanges.

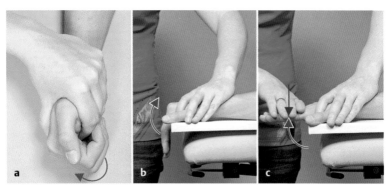

Fig. 125   Testing of extension in the metacarpophalangeal joints for grades 2, 3, 4, 5, and 6.

■ Flexion in the Metacarpophalangeal Joints (Fig. 126)

	Muscle	Origin	Insertion
	Interossei palmares muscles	Second, fourth, and fifth metacarpals	Bases of second, fourth, and fifth proximal phalanges and corresponding dorsal aponeuroses
	Ulnar nerve (C8–T1)		
1	*Dorsal interossei muscles*	Aspects of the five metacarpals that face each other	Bases of proximal phalanges, posterior aponeuroses of second to fifth fingers
	Ulnar nerve (C8–T1)		
2	*Lumbricals*	Radial side of flexor digitorum profundus tendons	Joint capsule of metacarpophalangeal joints, aponeuroses of extensors
	Median nerve, ulnar nerve (C8–T1)		
	Flexor digitorum superficialis muscle	Medial epicondyle of humerus, coronoid process, radius	Center of medial phalanges of second to fifth fingers
	Median nerve (C7–T1)		
	Flexor digitorum profundus muscle	Proximal two-thirds of palmar surface of ulna, interosseous membrane	Bases of distal phalanges of second to fifth fingers
	Anterior interosseous branch of the median nerve, ulnar nerve (C6–T1)		
	Flexor digiti minimi brevis muscle	Flexor retinaculum, hook of hamate bone	Palmar surface of base of proximal phalanx
	Ulnar nerve (C8–T1)		

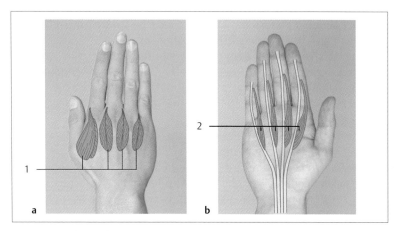

Fig. 126   Muscles involved in metacarpophalangeal joint flexion:
1   Dorsal interossei muscles
2   Lumbricals

Clinical Symptoms

Shortening: Extension is limited in all finger joints.

Shortening of the flexor digitorum superficialis and flexor digitorum profundus muscles becomes evident if finger extension is performed together with wrist extension.

Weakness: In addition to reduced strength during flexion of the metacarpophalangeal joint, weakness of the involved muscles also results in loss of strength during distal and proximal flexion of the interphalangeal joint, and during wrist flexion. For the patient, this means considerable functional loss, since he or she cannot make a good fist. Patients cannot maintain wrist flexion while lifting heavy objects.

If weakness during flexion in the metacarpophalangeal joints predominates, the interossei muscles and the lumbricals will be more strongly affected, since they are the strongest flexors of these joints. Clinically, symptoms resemble paresis of the ulnar nerve (see p. 256).

1. For palpation, the patient's forearm rests on the treatment table, in supination. The examiner stabilizes the wrist.
   The interossei palmares muscles cannot be palpated, since they are deep muscles and are covered by other muscles and tendons.
2. The patient's forearm rests on the treatment table, in a neutral position. The examiner stabilizes the wrist from the volar side (**Fig. 127 a**).
   The patient performs flexion of the metacarpophalangeal joint, over the full range of motion.
3. The patient's forearm rests on the treatment table, in supination. The examiner stabilizes the wrist (**Fig. 127 b**).
4. 5. 6. Starting position and stabilization are the same as for grade 3 (**Fig. 127 c**).
   The examiner applies resistance to the proximal phalanges.

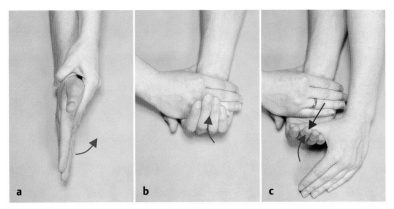

Fig. 127   Testing of flexion in the metacarpophalangeal joints for grades 2, 3, 4, 5, and 6.

■ Extension in the Proximal Interphalangeal and Distal Interphalangeal Joints (Fig. 128)

	Muscle	Origin	Insertion
1	*Extensor digitorum muscle* Radial nerve (C6–C8)	Lateral epicondyle of humerus, lateral collateral ligament, annular ligament of radius, antebrachial fascia	Posterior aponeuroses of second to fifth fingers
	Extensor indicis muscle Radial nerve (C6–C8)	Posterior surface of ulna, interosseous membrane	Posterior aponeurosis of index finger
	Extensor digiti minimi muscle Radial nerve (C6–C8)	Lateral epicondyle of humerus, lateral collateral ligament, annular ligament of radius	Posterior aponeurosis of fifth finger
	Interossei palmares muscles Ulnar nerve (C8–T1)	Second, fourth, and fifth metacarpals	Bases of proximal phalanges, posterior aponeuroses
2	*Dorsal interossei muscles* Ulnar nerve (C8–T1)	Two-headed from facing sides of the five metacarpals	Bases of proximal phalanges, posterior aponeuroses
	Lumbricals Median nerve, ulnar nerve (C8–T1)	Radial side of flexor digitorum profundus tendons	Joint capsule of metacarpophalangeal joints, posterior aponeuroses

Clinical Symptoms

Shortening: Flexion is restricted in all finger joints. Shortening becomes particularly evident when finger flexion is combined with wrist flexion and elbow extension. Persistent shortening can irritate the origin tendons at the lateral epicondyle.

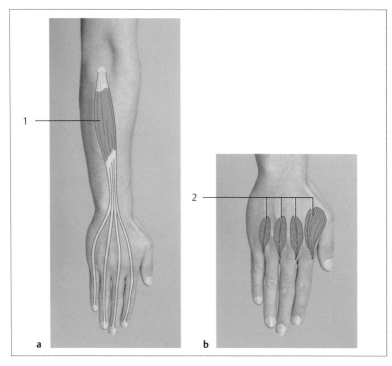

Fig. 128   Muscles involved in proximal and distal interphalangeal joint extension:
1   Extensor digitorum muscle
2   Dorsal interossei muscles

The examiner can detect shortening of the interossei muscles and the lumbricals if the metacarpophalangeal joints are extended and the proximal and distal interphalangeal joints flexed.

Weakness: Weakness clearly reduces strength during finger extension and during wrist extension.

If the interossei muscles and the lumbricals are affected, strength is reduced during flexion of the metacarpophalangeal joint and during finger spreading and closing.

1 The examiner palpates the muscles, with the patient's forearm resting on the treatment table in pronation. The examiner holds the hand and stabilizes the metacarpophalangeal joints in extension from the volar side.

   The interossei palmares muscles and the lumbricals are covered by other muscles and tendons, and cannot be palpated.

2 The patient's forearm rests pronated on the table and the medial and distal phalanges of the fingers are hanging over the edge of the treatment table. The examiner stabilizes the metacarpophalangeal joints (**Fig. 129 a**).

   The patient extends the proximal and distal interphalangeal joints over the first half of the range of motion.

3 Starting position and stabilization are the same as for evaluation of grade 2 muscle strength.

   Both joints are fully extended.

4 5 6 Starting position and stabilization are the same as for grade 2 (**Fig. 129 b**).

   The examiner applies resistance to the medial and proximal phalanges.

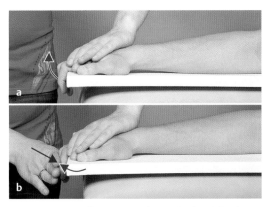

Fig. 129 Testing of extension in the proximal and distal interphalangeal joints for grades 2, 3, 4, 5, and 6.

■ Flexion in the Proximal Interphalangeal Joints (Fig. 130)

	Muscle	Origin	Insertion
1	*Flexor digitorum profundus muscle* Anterior interosseous branch of the median nerve, ulnar nerve (C6–T1)	Proximal two-thirds of palmar surface of ulna, interosseous membrane	Bases of distal phalanges of second to fifth fingers
2	*Flexor digitorum superficialis muscle* Median nerve (C7–T1)	Medial epicondyle of humerus, coronoid process, radius	Center of medial phalanges of second to fifth fingers

Clinical Symptoms

Shortening: Extension is limited in all finger joints, especially when combined with wrist extension.

Weakness: Strength is reduced both during distal and proximal flexion of the interphalangeal joint and during wrist flexion. The patient cannot maintain wrist flexion when lifting heavy objects.

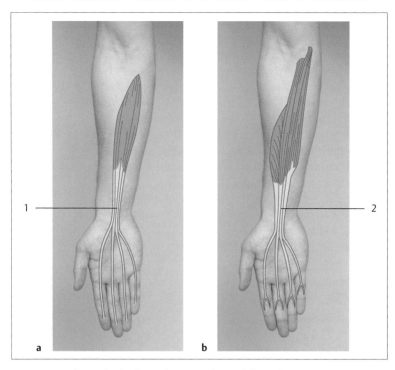

a b

Fig. 130 Muscles involved in flexing the proximal interphalangeal joints:
1 Flexor digitorum profundus muscle
2 Flexor digitorum superficialis muscle

1   The examiner palpates the muscle, with the patient's forearm resting on the treatment table in supination.

The examiner stabilizes the metacarpophalangeal joints, in extension (**Fig. 131** for grade 2).

2   The patient's forearm rests on the treatment table, in supination. The examiner stabilizes the metacarpophalangeal joints in extension (**Fig. 131 a**).

The patient performs up to half the range of motion for flexion in the proximal interphalangeal joints of the fingers.

3   Starting position and stabilization are the same as for evaluation of grade 2 muscle strength.

The patient performs the full range of motion.

4 5 6 Starting position and stabilization are the same as for grade 2 (**Fig. 131 b**).

The examiner applies resistance to the medial phalanges.

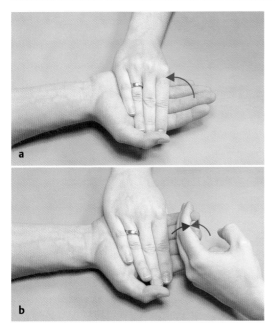

Fig. 131   Testing of flexion in the proximal interphalangeal joints for grades 2, 3, 4, 5, and 6.

■ Flexion in the Distal Interphalangeal Joints (Fig. 132)

	Muscle	Origin	Insertion
1	*Flexor digitorum profundus muscle*	Proximal two-thirds of palmar surface of ulna, interosseous membrane	Bases of distal phalanges of second to fifth fingers
	Anterior interosseous branch of the median nerve, ulnar nerve (C6–T1)		

Clinical Symptoms

Shortening: Extension is limited in all finger joints, especially when combined with wrist extension.

Weakness: Strength is reduced during finger and wrist flexion.

---

[1] For palpation, the patient's forearm rests on the treatment table, in supination. The examiner stabilizes the proximal interphalangeal joints in extension.

[2] The patient's forearm rests on the treatment table, in supination. The examiner stabilizes the proximal interphalangeal joints in extension.

The patient flexes the distal interphalangeal joints over part of the range of motion. The examiner performs the test for each joint individually.

[3] Starting position and stabilization are the same as for evaluation of grade 2 muscle strength.

The movement is executed fully.

[4] [5] [6] Starting position and stabilization are the same as for grade 2 (**Fig. 133**). The examiner applies resistance to the distal phalanx of the finger being tested.

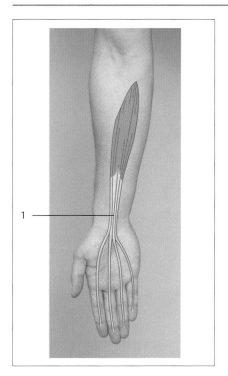

Fig. 132 Muscles involved in flexing the distal interphalangeal joints:
1 Flexor digitorum profundus muscle

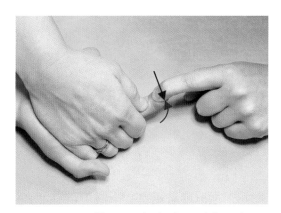

Fig. 133 Testing of flexion in the distal interphalangeal joints for grades 2, 3, 4, 5, and 6.

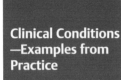

Clinical Conditions —Examples from Practice

Manual muscle testing of the upper extremity muscles was described in the previous section. This section describes the most significant forms of peripheral paralysis of the upper extremity and the forms that are most commonly observed in physical therapy practice.

Awareness of how these forms of paralysis present is very important for diagnosis and treatment.

In addition to functional loss, visible atrophy, compensatory movements, and secondary damage are present.

Winged Scapula due to Peripheral Nerve Damage

The following peripheral nerves may be affected:
- long thoracic nerve (C5–C7) (e.g., damage caused by lifting heavy loads)
- accessory nerve (cranial nerve with its own nucleus in the medulla oblongata; nucleus extends down to the level of C5–C6) (**Fig. 134**)
- dorsal scapular nerve (C4–C5) (e.g., in cases of brachial plexus injury).

Depending on which nerve has been damaged, the anterior serratus muscle (long thoracic nerve), the trapezius muscle (accessory nerve), or the rhomboid muscles (dorsal scapular nerve) will be affected. All three forms of paralysis will present clinically as winged scapula. However, the various combinations of paretic and intact muscles determine the different positions of the scapula medially and toward the thorax when at rest and while moving.

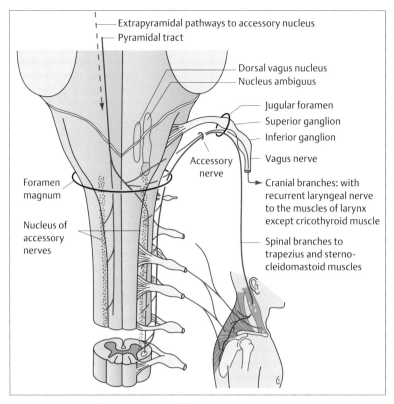

Fig. 134   Course and motor innervation of the accessory nerve.

If the forward and lateral pulling action of the *serratus anterior muscle* is lost, the scapula will be pulled medially by the trapezius and rhomboid muscles. The medial border of the scapula clearly protrudes from the rib cage. The patient is unable to elevate the arm through the full range of motion, because the trapezius muscle can only partially rotate the scapula. During the movement, scapular winging is exacerbated (**Fig. 135**).

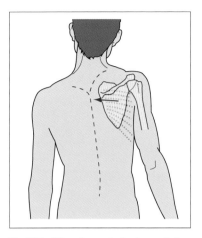

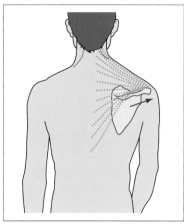

Fig. 135 Winged scapula due to paralysis of the serratus anterior muscle.

Fig. 136 Winged scapula due to paralysis of the trapezius muscle.

If the *trapezius muscle* is weakened due to accessory nerve damage, the scapula will move laterally and anteriorly toward the spinal column, owing to the action of the serratus anterior and pectoralis minor muscles. The medial border of the scapula will move away slightly from the rib cage; the patient compensates for this, in part, when lifting the arm, because of the action of the serratus anterior muscle. However, in this case also, the patient will not be able to fully elevate the arm (**Fig. 136**).

Winged scapula is least pronounced if it is caused by paralysis of the *rhomboid muscles*. In this case, the scapula will also move away somewhat from the spinal column in a lateral direction. However, the patient will be able to rotate the scapula completely via the serratus anterior and trapezius muscles, and will therefore be able to elevate the arm through the full range of motion (**Fig. 137**).

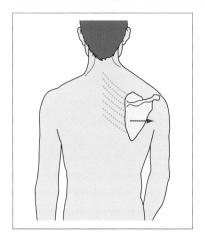

Fig. 137   Winged scapula due to paralysis of the rhomboid muscles.

Winged Scapula in Patients with Muscular Weakness

Abnormal posture with a strong kyphotic curvature in the thoracic spine usually occurs in combination with weak rhomboid and trapezius muscles.

The scapula deviates medially from the spinal column and protrudes from the rib cage. In many cases, the patient cannot achieve the full range of motion during arm elevation, and strength is reduced when lifting the arm. If the patient holds a light weight with the arms extended forward, the border of the scapula will detach itself from the rib cage after a short time (Matthiass I, II, III, see pp. 43 and 44).

This muscular deficit can bring about overuse symptoms of the active and passive stabilizing structures of the shoulder joint.

Erb Palsy

Erb palsy is generally caused by direct impact. It is frequently the result of motorcycle accidents or trauma at birth.

In this condition, the nerves from the C5 and C6 spinal cord segments and, less frequently, the C7 nerve, are damaged (Duus 2012).

The muscles innervated by these nerves can be weakened to varying degrees, depending on the injury site, since they are generally innervated by at least two nerves. The paresis primarily manifests itself in the following muscles:

Muscle	Innervation
Deltoid muscle	Axillary nerve (C4–C6)
Teres minor muscle	Axillary nerve (C4–C6)
Supraspinatus muscle	Suprascapular nerve (C4–C6)
Infraspinatus muscle	Suprascapular nerve (C4–C6)
Anterior serratus muscle	Long thoracic nerve (C5–C7)
Rhomboid muscles	Dorsal scapular nerve (C4–C5)
Biceps brachii muscle	Musculocutaneous nerve (C5–C6)
Brachioradialis muscle	Radial nerve (C5–C6)
Supinator muscle	Radial nerve (C5–C6)

Owing to the paralysis of the *deltoid, supraspinatus, infraspinatus, and teres minor muscles*, the patient's arm is internally rotated and hangs down flaccidly next to the body. The patient's shoulder is pulled forward and the medial border of the scapula protrudes from the rib cage, owing to paralysis of the *serratus anterior* and *rhomboid muscles,* as is typical for winged scapula.

Deltoid and biceps brachii atrophy will be clearly evident. The humeral head is subluxed, with a typical "dent" below the acromion (**Fig. 138**).

The most important functions lost due to Erb palsy are the ability to lift the arm forward and to the side, along with elbow flexion.

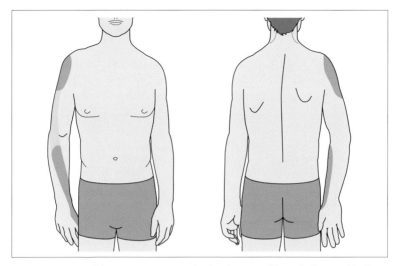

Fig. 138   Position of the arm in a patient with Erb palsy, viewed from the front and back.

The patient is unable to fully compensate for being unable to lift the arm by raising the shoulder and bending the trunk laterally.

There is sensory impairment over the deltoid muscle and on the radial side of the forearm and hand (**Fig. 138**, areas shaded red).

Klumpke Paralysis

In this condition, the C8–T1 spinal nerves and, in some cases, the C7 spinal nerve, are damaged (Duus 2012).

The paralysis affects the small hand muscles and finger flexors; the wrist flexors are not affected as often. There is sensory impairment in the area of the ulnar nerve.

Owing to the dominance of the extensors and paralysis of the *interosseous muscles* and *lumbricals* (extension in the proximal and distal interphalangeal joints of the fingers), the hand is in a claw position.

Suprascapular Nerve Palsy (C4–C6)

Suprascapular nerve palsy affects the supraspinatus and infraspinatus muscles. In addition to abducting the shoulder joint, the *supraspinatus muscle* works as a joint-stabilizing muscle. Paralysis of this muscle affects abduction. The deltoid muscle can, for the most part, perform the movement alone, but the movement will lack strength. The joint-stabilizing function consists of contracting the cranial part of the shoulder capsule and pressing the humeral head into the socket during abduction. Owing to the loss of this joint-stabilizing function, paralysis can result in overloading of other shoulder muscles, such as the long head of the biceps brachii, subscapularis, or teres minor muscles. A deficit of the *infraspinatus muscle* leads to substantial loss of strength during external rotation in the shoulder joint, since only the teres minor muscle and the posterior part of the deltoid muscle can then perform this movement. Together with the teres minor muscle, the infraspinatus muscle acts to tighten the posterior capsule. They prevent the humeral head from dislocating posteriorly. Paralysis of the infraspinatus muscle will result in overloading of other shoulder joint muscles, such as the subscapularis muscle and/or teres minor muscle (**Fig. 139**).

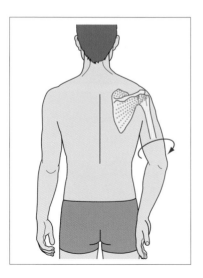

Fig. 139   Position of the arm in a patient with suprascapular nerve palsy.

If the palsy persists for a long time, atrophy of the infraspinatus muscle below the scapular spine will be clearly evident. Any atrophy of the supraspinatus muscle will not be as obvious because this muscle is covered by the trapezius muscle.

Axillary Nerve Palsy (C4–C6)

In most cases, the nerve is damaged as a result of shoulder dislocation, humerus fractures, or pressure from crutches.

The *deltoid* and *teres minor muscles* are affected, significantly weakening forward flexion and abduction of the arm, and considerably reducing external rotation strength.

The patient can only partially abduct the arm via the supraspinatus muscle and can only partially lift the arm via the long head of the biceps brachii, coracobrachialis, and pectoralis major muscles. The infraspinatus muscle is still available to perform external rotation of the arm.

However, reduced strength is clearly evident in all three movements.

If the palsy persists for a long time, the change in the shoulder profile due to the atrophy of the deltoid muscle becomes evident. The shoulder becomes flatter and the acromion protrudes at an angle.

The lack of muscle stabilization causes hyperextension of the contractile and non-contractile structures; this, in turn, causes shoulder subluxation or even dislocation (**Fig. 140**).

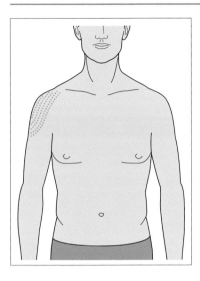

Fig. 140   Axillary nerve palsy.

Musculocutaneous Nerve Palsy (C5–C6)

The musculocutaneous nerve innervates the *biceps brachii, brachialis*, and *coracobrachialis muscles.* Elbow flexion is the primary function affected. The brachioradialis, pronator teres, flexor carpi radialis, and flexor carpi ulnaris muscles, the humeral head of the flexor digitorum superficialis muscle, and the wrist extensors can only perform the movement very weakly and cannot perform the full range of motion. The arm can still be elevated using the deltoid and pectoralis major (clavicular and sternal parts) muscles, albeit more weakly.

The strength of forearm supination is substantially reduced, owing to the paralysis of the biceps brachii muscle. Flattening of the shoulder profile in the area of the upper arm flexors and complete extension of the arm hanging down is striking (**Fig. 141**).

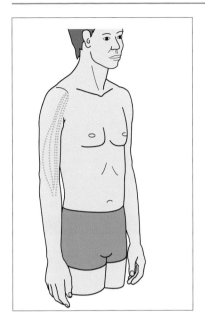

Fig. 141   Musculocutaneous nerve palsy.

Radial Nerve Palsy (C5–C8)

The clinical presentation of radial nerve palsy always depends on the injury site, since the motor branches leave the nerve at the upper arm and forearm at various levels. For example, if there is axillary damage, all of the muscles innervated by the radial nerve will be affected. These muscles are the *triceps brachii, brachioradialis*, and *supinator muscles*, all of the *finger* and *wrist extensors*, as well as the *abductor pollicis longus muscle*. This means that elbow extension will be completely absent, elbow flexion will be somewhat weaker, supination strength will be considerably reduced, and forearm pronation strength up to neutral position will also be reduced. The wrist and finger joints cannot be actively extended. If the nerve is damaged at the upper arm, distal to where it branches off to the triceps brachii muscle, elbow extension will be intact. If the injury site is at the forearm, the finger and wrist extensors will also be paralyzed. Wrist drop is a typical sign of radial nerve palsy, regardless of the injury site (**Fig. 142**).

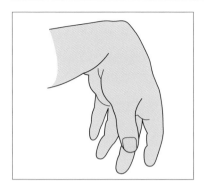

Fig. 142   Wrist drop in a patient with radial nerve palsy.

Ulnar Nerve Palsy (C8–T1)

Ulnar nerve palsy primarily manifests itself by paralysis of the interossei muscles and the ensuing claw hand. Additional symptoms include the paralysis of both ulnar lumbrical muscles, the deep head of the flexor pollicis brevis muscle, the adductor pollicis muscle, and the muscles of the hypothenar eminence. If the damage occurs in the elbow area, the flexor carpi ulnaris, palmaris longus, and fourth and fifth finger flexor digitorum profundus muscles will also be affected. The claw hand that is typical of ulnar nerve palsy can be explained by the paralysis of the aforementioned muscles and the ensuing dominance of the opposing muscles. Hyperextension in the metacarpophalangeal joints is particularly striking, especially in the fourth and fifth fingers (**Fig. 143**). Ulnar nerve palsy is often caused by direct trauma or by pressure in the area of the ulnar groove.

The interosseous muscles and lumbricals have the greatest impact on flexion of the metacarpophalangeal joints. As a result, when these muscles are paralyzed, the finger extensors dominate in the metacarpophalangeal joints. The second and third fingers are less affected by this hyperextension because the two lumbricals and all the long finger flexors are still functional in this scenario.

The thumb is abducted and hyperextended in the metacarpophalangeal joint. Paralysis of the adductor pollicis muscle causes dominance of the thumb abductors and weakness of the short head of the flexor pollicis

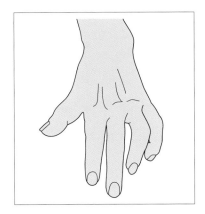

Fig. 143 Claw hand in a patient with ulnar nerve palsy.

brevis muscle, which in turn causes the extensors to hyperextend the metacarpophalangeal joint.

Paralysis of the adductor pollicis muscle leads to a positive *Froment sign*: When the patient attempts to hold a sheet of paper with the pincer grip, he or she compensates for the ensuing muscle weakness by using the flexor pollicis longus muscle, which, in turn, causes the thumb interphalangeal joint to flex.

In the case of long-term palsy, atrophy between the metacarpal bones and at the hypothenar eminence is clearly evident.

Median Nerve Palsy (C5–T1)

High-level paralysis of the median nerve leads to the characteristic ape hand deformity. The wrist joint is extended because the *flexor digitorum superficialis* and the *flexor digitorum profundus muscles* for the second and third fingers, as well as the *flexor carpi radialis muscle*, are paralyzed. The thumb, index, and middle fingers are extended, owing to the weakness of the *flexor pollicis longus, flexor digitorum superficialis*, and *flexor digitorum profundus muscles* (second and third fingers) and the two medial lumbricals. In addition, the thumb lies flat against the index finger, since the *abductor pollicis brevis* and *opponens pollicis muscles* and the *superficial head of the flexor pollicis brevis muscle* are also affected (**Fig. 144**).

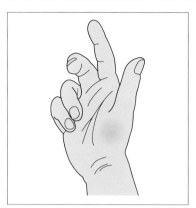

Fig. 144 "Ape hand deformity" in a patient with median nerve palsy.

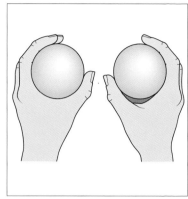

Fig. 145 The right hand has a positive bottle sign, which is caused by median nerve palsy.

If the median nerve is damaged distal to the mid-forearm, only the small hand muscles innervated by the median nerve will be paralyzed.

In both cases, if the palsy persists for a long time, it will lead to clear atrophy of the thenar eminence ("ape hand"). In both cases, the *bottle sign* will also be positive. If the patient attempts to grasp a glass or a bottle with the affected hand, he or she will be unable to sufficiently abduct the thumb; as a consequence, the web between the thumb and index finger will not touch the object (**Fig. 145**).

The thumb's opposition movement is impaired. It can only be partially performed by flexing the distal interphalangeal joint. Thumb pronator rotation is completely absent. The palsy is usually caused by trauma or by pressure lesions (e.g., "Saturday night palsy"). It is frequently caused by narrowing of the median nerve in the carpal tunnel.

6
Lower Extremity

Muscles and Manual Muscle Testing of the Lower Extremity

Hip Joint

■ Extension at the Hip (Fig. 146)

	Muscle	Origin	Insertion
1	Gluteus maximus muscle	Iliac crest, posterior superior iliac spine, thoracolumbar fascia, sacrum, coccyx, wing of ilium	Iliotibial tract, gluteal tuberosity
	Inferior gluteal nerve (L5–S2)		
2	Semitendinosus muscle	Ischial tuberosity	Superficial pes anserinus
3	Semimembranosus muscle	Ischial tuberosity	Medial condyle of tibia, joint capsule
	Tibial nerve (L5–S2)		
4	Gluteus medius muscle (posterior part)	Gluteal surface of wing of ilium	Greater trochanter
5	Gluteus minimus muscle (posterior part)	Gluteal surface of wing of ilium	Greater trochanter
	Superior gluteal nerve (L4–S1)		
6	Adductor magnus muscle	Inferior ramus of pubis, ramus of ischium, ischial tuberosity	Medial lip of linea aspera, adductor tubercle of medial epicondyle
	Obturator nerve (L2–L4), tibial nerve (L3–L5)		
7	Biceps femoris muscle (long head) Tibial nerve (L5–S2)	Ischial tuberosity	Head of fibula

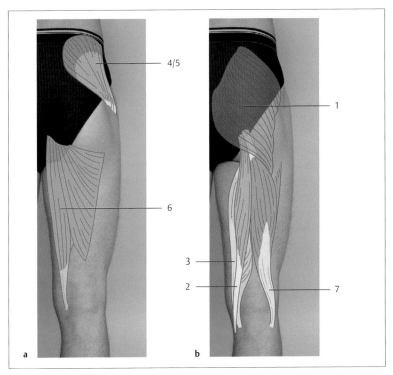

Fig. 146 Muscles involved in extension at the hip:

1	Gluteus maximus muscle
2	Semitendinosus muscle
3	Semimembranosus muscle
4/5	Gluteus medius and minimus muscles
6	Adductor magnus muscle
7	Biceps femoris muscle

Clinical Symptoms

Shortening: Shortening of the gluteus maximus muscle is rare. Contractures of the other muscles are described under their primary functions.

Weakness: The patient is unsteady during the stance phase and compensates for this weakness by bending the upper body backward; this, in turn, passively extends the hip joint. The iliofemoral ligament limits hyperextension in the hip joint and provides the patient with passive ligament-induced stability (see pp. 329 and 330).

1. The examiner palpates the gluteus maximus muscle, with the patient prone. It is easiest to contract this muscle when the spine is extended. The following muscles, which participate in hip extension, will be easier to palpate when they are actively performing their primary action:
   - gluteus medius and minimus muscles (hip abduction, see pp. 270 and 271),
   - adductor magnus muscle (hip adduction, see pp. 274 and 275)
   - semitendinosus muscle (knee flexion, see pp. 292 and 293)
   - semimembranosus muscle (knee flexion, see pp. 292 and 293)
   - biceps femoris muscle (knee flexion, see pp. 292 and 293).

2. The test is performed with the patient lying on one side (**Fig. 147 a**). The examiner holds the upper leg in slight abduction and flexion, in order to prevent lordosis in the lumbar spine during the movement. The bottom leg (the one being tested) is in maximum hip flexion.
   The movement is performed with approximately 80° to 90° knee flexion, to prevent the patient from simulating the movement by extending the knee.
   The patient must be prevented from making compensatory movements with the upper body.

3. The patient is prone (**Fig. 147 b**), with the legs off the table. The patient stands on the leg not being tested, beside the table, to stabilize the pelvis. The examiner also stabilizes the pelvis. The movement is performed with the knee of the patient's free leg slightly flexed.

4. 5. 6. Starting position and stabilization are the same as for grade 3 (**Fig. 147 c**).
   The examiner applies resistance to the back of the lower third of the thigh.

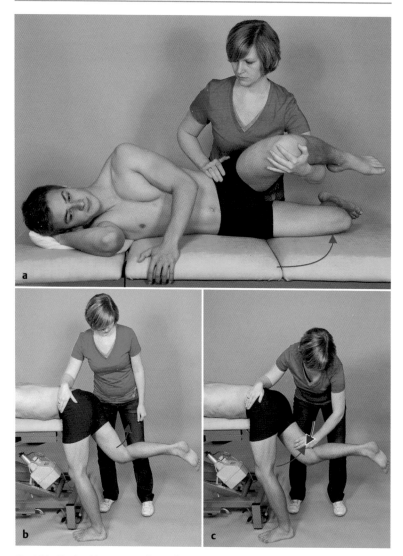

Fig. 147   Testing hip extension for grades 2, 3, 4, 5, and 6.

■ Flexion at the Hip (Fig. 148)

	Muscle	Origin	Insertion
1	*Iliopsoas muscle*		
	Psoas major muscle	Lateral surfaces of T12 and L1–L4 vertebrae and the intervertebral disks located between them, costal processes of L1–L5 vertebrae	Lesser trochanter
	Iliacus muscle	Iliac fossa, region of anterior inferior iliac spine	Lesser trochanter
	Lumbar plexus, femoral nerve (psoas major muscle L1–L3, iliacus muscle L2–L4)		
2	*Rectus femoris muscle* Femoral nerve (L2–L4)	Anterior inferior iliac spine, superior border of acetabulum	Tibial tuberosity
3	*Tensor of fascia lata muscle* Superior gluteal nerve (L4–L5)	Anterior superior iliac spine	Iliotibial tract (lateral condyle of tibia)
4	*Sartorius muscle* Femoral nerve (L1–L3)	Anterior superior iliac spine	Superficial pes anserinus
	Gluteus minimus muscle (anterior part) Superior gluteal nerve (L4–L5)	Gluteal surface of wing of ilium	Greater trochanter
	Gluteus medius muscle (anterior part) Superior gluteal nerve (L4–S1)	Gluteal surface of wing of ilium	Greater trochanter
	Pectineus muscle Femoral nerve (L2–L3) Obturator nerve (L2–L4)	Pecten pubis	Pubic tubercle

Muscle	Origin	Insertion
Adductor longus muscle Obturator nerve (L2–L4)	Superior ramus of pubis	Medial lip of linea aspera
Adductor magnus muscle Obturator nerve (L2–L4) Tibial nerve (L3–L5)	Inferior ramus of pubis, ramus of ischium, ischial tuberosity	Medial lip of linea aspera, adductor tubercle of medial epicondyle
Adductor brevis muscle Obturator nerve (L2–L4)	Inferior ramus of pubis	Medial lip of linea aspera
Gracilis muscle Obturator nerve (L2–L4)	Inferior ramus of pubis	Superficial pes anserinus

Clinical Symptoms

Shortening: Shortening of the hip flexors causes pelvic tilt, exaggerated lumbar lordosis, and limited hip joint extension.

If there is unilateral shortening (see pp. 330 and 331), the ilium on the affected side will be tilted forward and the ilium on the non-affected side will remain in its anatomical position. This may result in pelvic twisting, with ensuing functional impairment in the lumbar, pelvic, and hip regions. If the shortening is bilateral (especially of the rectus femoris muscle and tensor of fascia lata muscle), the pelvic tilt will become more pronounced, which can, in turn, overload the lumbosacral transitional vertebrae.

Weakness: During gait, the patient uses circumduction in the hip joint to bring the leg forward.

It is nearly impossible for the patient to climb stairs unaided. Despite intact abdominal muscles, the patient is unable to get into a sitting position from the supine position without using the arms for support, since the hip joint (pelvis = mobile attachment, thigh = fixed attachment) cannot be flexed with enough force.

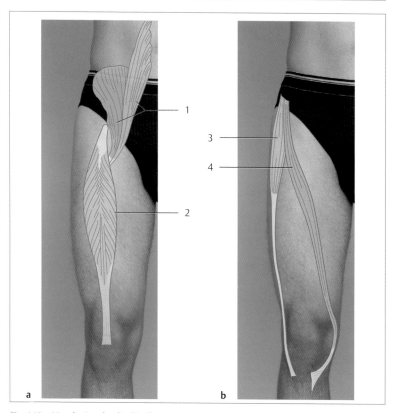

Fig. 148   Muscles involved in hip flexion:
1   Iliopsoas muscle
2   Rectus femoris muscle
3   Tensor of fascia lata muscle
4   Sartorius muscle

1. Palpation is performed with the patient supine, with the examiner holding the leg with the hip and knee slightly flexed.
   The following muscles, which participate in hip flexion, will be easier to palpate when they are actively performing their primary action:
   - rectus femoris muscle (knee extension, see pp. 288 and 289)
   - gluteus medius and minimus muscles (hip abduction, see pp. 270 and 271)
   - pectineus muscle (hip adduction, see pp. 274 and 275)
   - adductor longus, magnus, and brevis muscles (hip adduction, see pp. 274 and 275)
   - gracilis muscle (hip adduction, see pp. 274 and 275).
2. The patient lies on one side (**Fig. 149 a**). The examiner stabilizes the pelvis and holds the upper part of the leg in slight abduction. The bottom leg (the one being tested) is fully extended at the hip joint. The knee is flexed approximately 80°, to prevent contraction in the hamstring muscles during the movement.
3. The patient is supine and the lower leg of the test leg hangs over the end of the treatment table (**Fig. 149 b**). The patient bends the knee of the leg not being tested and places the foot on the table to prevent exaggerated lumbar lordosis. If the patient is able to flex the hip joint in this position up to a 90° angle, the movement receives grade 2–3. For grade 3, the examiner tests hip flexion with the patient sitting at the edge of the table (90° hip flexion). The patient must avoid leaning the upper body backward; otherwise spinal flexion will mask the hip flexion movement (**Fig. 149 c**).
4. 5. 6. The patient sits at the end of the treatment table. The examiner applies resistance above the patient's knee (**Fig. 149 d**).

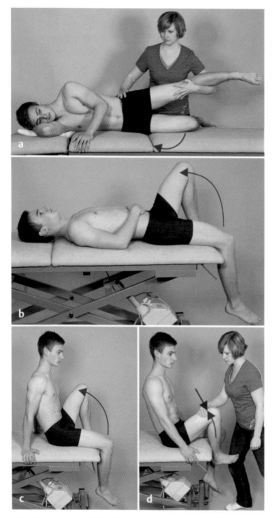

Fig. 149   Testing of hip flexion for grades 2, 3, 4, 5, and 6.

■ Abduction at the Hip (Fig. 150)

	Muscle	Origin	Insertion
1	*Gluteus medius muscle* Superior gluteal nerve (L4–L5)	Gluteal surface of wing of ilium	Greater trochanter
2	*Tensor of fascia lata muscle* Superior gluteal nerve (L4–L5)	Anterior superior iliac spine	Iliotibial tract, lateral condyle of tibia
3	*Gluteus maximus muscle (iliotibial tract)* Inferior gluteal nerve (L5–L2)	Iliac crest, posterior superior iliac spine	Iliotibial tract
	Gluteus minimus muscle Superior gluteal nerve (L4–S1)	Gluteal surface of wing of ilium	Greater trochanter
	Rectus femoris muscle Femoral nerve (L2–L4)	Anterior inferior iliac spine, superior border of acetabulum	Tibial tuberosity
	Piriformis muscle Sacral plexus (L5–S2)	Pelvic surface of sacrum	Medial side of greater trochanter

Clinical Symptoms

Shortening: The pelvis is tilted toward the shortened side. The leg on the affected side is functionally longer (see pp. 332 and 333). The patient compensates for the discrepancy by flexing the hip and knee or by abducting the affected leg.

The joints of the lower extremity and the lumbar, pelvic, and hip regions are improperly loaded. This pathological loading can result in overloading of all involved structures and can cause functional impairment in the motion of spinal segments or the sacro-iliac joints.

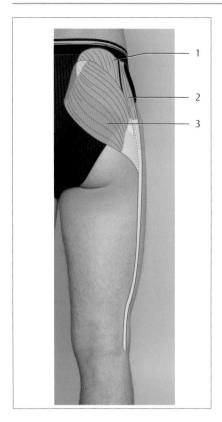

Fig. 150 Muscles involved in hip abduction:
1   Gluteus medius and minimus muscles
2   Tensor of fascia lata muscle
3   Gluteus maximus muscle

Weakness: Lack of muscular stability means that the pelvis cannot be held on the weakened side during the stance phase and the other side drops (Trendelenburg sign). If there is bilateral weakness, the "catwalk gait pattern" can be observed.

Another type of compensation involves the patient bending the upper body to the side of the supporting leg, to prevent the pelvis from dropping (Duchenne sign), described as "waddling gait" (see pp. 332–335).

☐1 The patient lies supine. The examiner palpates the gluteus medius and minimus muscles at the lateral side of the pelvis above the greater trochanter and palpates the tensor of fascia lata muscle below the anterior superior iliac spine. The piriformis muscle cannot be palpated because it is covered by the gluteus maximus muscle.
The following muscles, which participate in hip flexion, will be easier to palpate when they are actively performing their primary action:
- gluteus maximus muscle (hip extension, see pp. 260 and 261)
- rectus femoris muscle (knee extension, see pp. 288 and 289).

☐2 Testing is performed with the patient supine (**Fig. 151 a**). The examiner stabilizes the pelvis on both sides, at the anterior superior iliac spine. The examiner places a cloth under the patient's heel, to reduce friction. If the abductors are weak, the patient can externally rotate the hip to use the flexors and simulate an abduction movement. The examiner can prevent this compensatory movement by asking the patient to initiate the movement from the heel.

☐3 The patient lies on one side, with the hip joints extended (**Fig. 151 b**).
The examiner stabilizes the pelvis. The patient is again asked to initiate the abduction movement from the heel.

☐4 ☐5 ☐6 Starting position and stabilization are the same as for grade 3 (**Fig. 151 c**).
The examiner applies resistance to the lateral side of the lower third of the thigh.

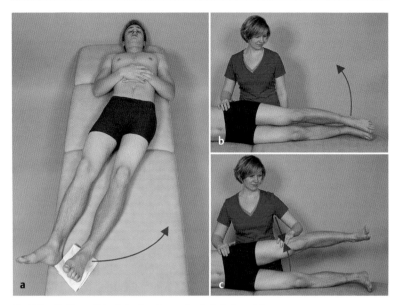

Fig. 151   Testing of hip abduction for grades 2, 3, 4, 5, and 6.

■ Adduction at the Hip (Fig. 152)

	Muscle	Origin	Insertion
1	*Adductor brevis muscle*	Inferior ramus of pubis	Medial lip of linea aspera
	Adductor longus muscle	Superior ramus of pubis	Medial lip of linea aspera
	Obturator nerve (L2–L4)		
	Adductor magnus muscle	Inferior ramus of pubis, ramus of ischium, ischial tuberosity	Medial lip of linea aspera, adductor tubercle of medial epicondyle of femur
	Obturator nerve (L2–L4) Tibial nerve (L3–L5)		
2	*Gluteus maximus muscle*	Iliac crest, posterior superior iliac spine, thoracolumbar fascia, sacrum, coccyx	Gluteal tuberosity of femur
	Inferior gluteal nerve (L5–S2)		
3 a	*Semitendinosus muscle*	Ischial tuberosity	Medial border of tibial tuberosity
3 b	*Semimembranosus muscle*	Ischial tuberosity	Medial condyle of tibia, joint capsule, oblique popliteal ligament
	Tibial nerve (L5–S2)		
4	*Biceps femoris muscle* (long head)	Ischial tuberosity	Head of fibula
	Tibial nerve (L5–S2)		
5	*Gracilis muscle*	Inferior ramus of pubis	Superficial pes anserinus
	Obturator nerve (L2–L4)		
6	*Pectineus muscle*	Pecten pubis	Pectineal line
	Femoral nerve, obturator nerve (L2–L4)		

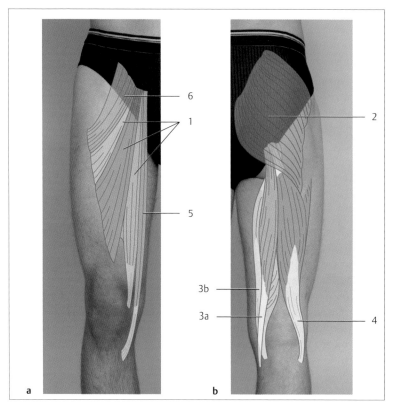

Fig. 152   Muscles involved in adducting the hip joint:

1   Adductor brevis, adductor longus, and adductor magnus muscles
2   Gluteus maximus muscle (inferior part)
3a   Semitendinosus muscle
3b   Semimembranosus muscle
4   Biceps femoris muscle
5   Gracilis muscle
6   Pectineus muscle

Clinical Symptoms

Shortening: Shortening of the hip adductors causes the leg on the affected side to be functionally shorter (see p. 332). The patient can compensate for this by:

- flexing the hip and knee of the non-affected leg
- abducting the non-affected leg.

As with abductor contracture, there is non-physiological loading that can place strain on individual structures. This frequently causes functional disturbances in the motion of lumbar segments, sacro-iliac joints, and joints of the lower extremity.

Weakness: Hip adductor weakness manifests itself in situations where the strength that needs to be exerted in the upper body must be transferred to the ground, for instance, when lifting heavy objects or when pulling or pushing heavy objects. This means that the patient will lack some stability during the stance phase and will not be able to produce full strength. The weakness is also noticeable when patients participate in sports such as horseback riding or skiing.

[1] The examiner palpates the adductor brevis, longus, and magnus muscles, and the gracilis and pectineus muscles on the medial thigh, with the patient supine. The following muscles, which participate in hip adduction, will be easier to palpate when they are actively performing their primary action:
- gluteus maximus muscle (hip extension, see pp. 260–263)
- semimembranosus muscle (knee flexion, see pp. 292–295)
- biceps femoris muscle (knee flexion, see pp. 292–295).

[2] Testing is performed with the patient supine (**Fig. 153a**). The examiner can stabilize the pelvis at both the anterior and superior iliac spines. The patient adducts the leg without rotating the hip joint. The examiner places a cloth under the patient's heel, to reduce friction.

[3] The patient lies on one side, with the hip joints extended (**Fig. 153b**).
The examiner holds the top leg in abduction and stabilizes the pelvis to prevent hip flexion. The patient raises the bottom leg. Hip extension must be maintained during the movement.

[4] [5] [6] Starting position and stabilization are the same as for grade 3 (**Fig. 153c**).
The examiner applies resistance to the medial side of the lower third of the thigh.

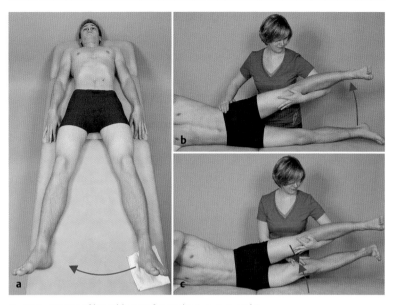

Fig. 153 Testing of hip adduction for grades 2, 3, 4, 5, and 6.

■ External Rotation at the Hip (Fig. 154)

	Muscle	Origin	Insertion
1	*Gluteus maximus muscle* Inferior gluteal nerve (L5–S2)	Iliac crest, posterior superior iliac spine, thoracolumbar fascia, sacrum, coccyx	Gluteal tuberosity, iliotibial tract
2	*Gluteus medius muscle (posterior part)* Superior gluteal nerve (L4–L5)	Gluteal surface of wing of ilium	Greater trochanter
3	*Gluteus minimus muscle (posterior part)* Superior gluteal nerve (L4–S1)	Gluteal surface of wing of ilium	Greater trochanter
4	*Iliopsoas muscle* *Psoas major muscle*	Lateral surfaces of T12 and L1–L4 vertebrae, along with the intervertebral disks located between them, costal processes of L1–L5 vertebrae	Lesser trochanter
	Iliacus muscle Lumbar plexus, femoral nerve (psoas major muscle L1–L3, iliacus muscle L2–L4)	Iliac fossa, region of anterior inferior iliac spine	Lesser trochanter
	Gemellus superior muscle	Ischial spine	Trochanteric fossa
	Gemellus inferior muscle Inferior gluteal nerve, sacral plexus (L5–S2)	Ischial tuberosity	Trochanteric fossa

	Muscle	Origin	Insertion
	Obturator internus muscle	Medial surface of hip bone around obturator foramen	Trochanteric fossa
	Inferior gluteal nerve, sacral plexus (L5–S2)		
	Piriformis muscle	Pelvic surface of sacrum, greater sciatic notch	Greater trochanter
	Sacral plexus (L5–S2)		
5	*Adductor magnus muscle*	Inferior ramus of pubis, ramus of ischium, ischial tuberosity	Medial lip of linea aspera
	Tibial nerve (L3–L5), obturator nerve (L2–L4)		
	Rectus femoris muscle	Anterior inferior iliac spine, superior border of acetabulum	Tibial tuberosity
	Femoral nerve (L2–L4)		
	Obturator externus muscle	Lateral surface of the medial border of obturator foramen, obturator membrane	Trochanteric fossa, joint capsule
	Obturator nerve (L2–L4)		
6	*Quadratus femoris muscle*	Ischial tuberosity	Intertrochanteric crest
	Inferior gluteal nerve, sacral plexus (L5–S2)		

Clinical Symptoms

Shortening: When the hip external rotators are shortened, the leg is externally rotated during loading and unloading.

Shortening of the short external rotators, in particular, can lead to functional disturbances in the sacro-iliac joints, owing to the unilateral traction at the sacrum.

Weakness: Weak hip external rotators will manifest themselves as internal rotation of the legs.

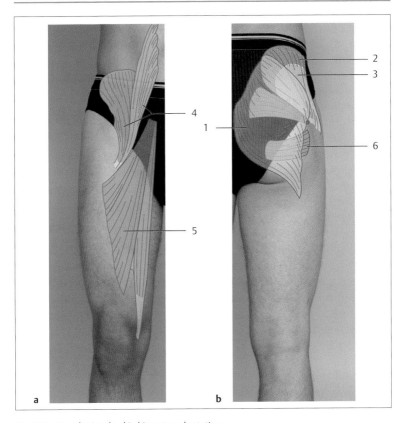

Fig. 154 Muscles involved in hip external rotation:
1 Gluteus maximus muscle
2 Gluteus medius muscle
3 Gluteus minimus muscle
4 Iliopsoas muscle
5 Adductor magnus muscle
6 Quadratus femoris muscle

1. The muscles of the hip joint that are predominantly external rotators are the obturator internus and externus muscles and the gemellus, quadratus femoris, and piriformis muscles.

   Since these muscles are covered by the gluteus maximus muscle, they are nearly impossible to palpate separately. It may be possible to palpate them if the gluteus maximus muscle is not innervated. The other participating muscles will be easier to palpate when they are actively performing their primary action:
   - gluteus maximus muscle (hip extension, see pp. 260 and 261)
   - gluteus medius and minimus muscles (hip abduction, see pp. 270 and 271)
   - iliopsoas muscle (hip flexion, see pp. 264 and 265)
   - adductor magnus muscle (hip adduction, see pp. 274 and 275)
   - rectus femoris muscle (knee extension, see pp. 288 and 289).

2. The patient is seated with the legs extended (**Fig. 155 a**). The examiner stabilizes the hemipelvis on the side being tested. The examiner exerts slight manual resistance against the gravity that arises from the movement starting from the neutral position.

3. The patient sits at the edge of the treatment table (**Fig. 155 b**). The examiner stabilizes the hemipelvis on the side opposite to the side being tested. The patient executes the movement from the neutral position to external rotation. The patient's thigh must remain on the table during the entire movement.

4. 5. 6. Starting position and stabilization are the same as for grade 3 (**Fig. 155 c**).

   The examiner exerts resistance near the knee on the lateral side of the thigh, as well as above the medial malleolus on the medial lower leg.

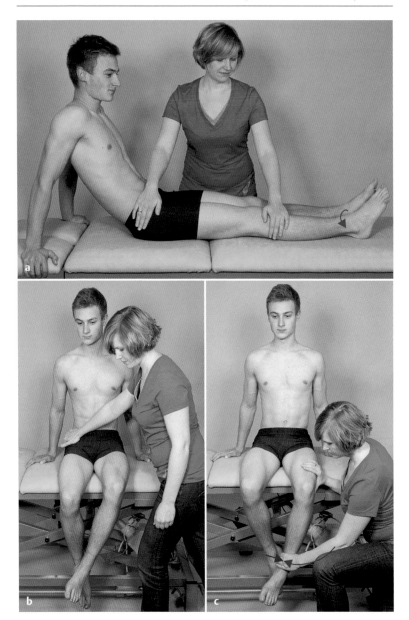

Fig. 155   Testing of hip external rotation for grades 2, 3, 4, 5, and 6.

■ Internal Rotation at the Hip (Fig. 156)

	Muscle	Origin	Insertion
1	Gluteus minimus muscle (anterior part) Superior gluteal nerve (L4–S1)	Lateral surface of ischium	Greater trochanter
2	Gluteus medius muscle (anterior part) Superior gluteal nerve (L4–L5)	Lateral surface of ischium	Greater trochanter
3	Tensor of fascia lata muscle Superior gluteal nerve (L4–L5)	Anterior superior iliac spine	Iliotibial tract (lateral condyle of tibia)
	Adductor magnus muscle Tibial nerve (L3–L5), obturator nerve (L2–L4)	Inferior ramus of pubis, ramus of ischium, ischial tuberosity	Adductor tubercle (medial epicondyle)

Clinical Symptoms

Since all the muscles that internally rotate the hip have other primary functions, **shortening** and, in particular, **weakness** of these muscles tend to be noticeable when they are performing their primary functions.

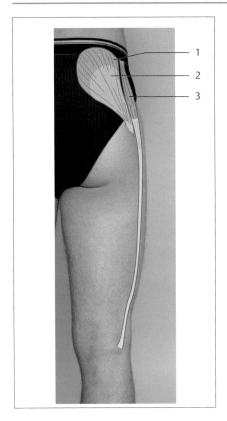

Fig. 156   Muscles involved in hip internal rotation:
1   Gluteus minimus muscle
2   Gluteus medius muscle
3   Tensor of fascia lata muscle

[1] It is easiest to palpate the internal rotators of the hip with the patient sitting with his or her legs extended.

All of the muscles involved in this function have another primary function. Therefore, if the examiner is unsure about a specific muscle's innervation, it should be evaluated when it is performing its primary function:

- gluteus medius and minimus muscles (hip abduction, see pp. 270 and 271)
- tensor of fascia lata muscle (hip abduction, see pp. 270 and 271)
- adductor magnus muscle (hip adduction, see pp. 274 and 275).

[2] The patient sits with the legs extended (**Fig. 157 a**). The examiner stabilizes the hemipelvis on the side being tested.

[3] The patient sits at the edge of the treatment table (**Fig. 157 b**). The examiner stabilizes the hemipelvis on the side being tested. The patient executes the movement from a neutral position to internal rotation.

[4] [5] [6] Starting position and stabilization are the same as for grade 3 (**Fig. 157 c**).

The examiner exerts resistance near the knee on the medial thigh and laterally above the lateral malleolus.

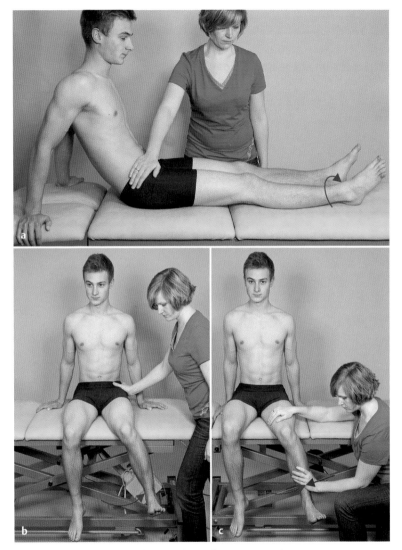

Fig. 157   Testing of hip internal rotation for grades 2, 3, 4, 5, and 6.

Knee Joint

■ Extension at the Knee (Fig. 158)

	Muscle	Origin	Insertion
1	Quadriceps femoris		
	Rectus femoris muscle	Anterior inferior iliac spine, superior border of acetabulum	Tibial tuberosity
	Vastus lateralis muscle	Lateral lip of linea aspera, lateral surface of greater trochanter, intertrochanteric line, gluteal tuberosity	Tibial tuberosity
	Vastus medialis muscle	Medial lip of linea aspera	Tibial tuberosity
	Vastus intermedius muscle	Anterior and lateral surface of femur	Tibial tuberosity
	Femoral nerve (L2–L4)		

The final degrees of knee extension are supported by tensor of fascia lata muscle activation.

2	Tensor of fascia lata muscle	Anterior superior iliac spine	Iliotibial tract (lateral condyle of tibia)
	Superior gluteal nerve (L4–L5)		

Clinical Symptoms

Shortening: If the quadriceps femoris is shortened, the rectus femoris muscle, as the only bi-articular component of the quadriceps femoris, is most noticeably affected. This shortening is clearly evident when the patient simultaneously extends the hip and flexes the knee. In this case, if there is a contracture, the patient will be unable to flex the knee completely or will be unable to extend the hip. The patient will compensate for the inability to extend the hip by increasing lumbar lordosis.

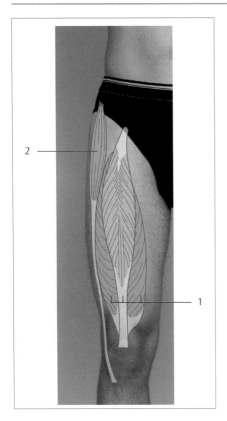

Fig. 158   Muscles involved in knee extension:
1   Quadriceps femoris muscle
2   Tensor of fascia lata muscle

Weakness: The patient will compensate for a weak quadriceps femoris by hyperextending the knee joint (genu recurvatum), to provide passive capsular stability when standing (see pp. 335 and 336).

During everyday activities, weakness is noticeable when climbing stairs and walking up inclines. The patient will place the hands on the knees for support when sitting down or standing up.

[1] The examiner palpates the quadriceps femoris, with its three components, the vastus lateralis, vastus medialis, and rectus femoris muscles, with the patient supine and the knee slightly flexed.
The vastus intermedius muscle is located below the rectus femoris muscle and cannot be palpated.

[2] The patient lies on one side (**Fig. 159 a**).
The examiner holds the patient's top leg in slight abduction. The bottom test leg is flexed at the hip and knee. The examiner stabilizes the leg at the thigh, to prevent the patient from simulating knee extension by flexing or extending the hip.

[3] The patient is supine, with the knee of the test leg bent and the lower leg hanging over the end of the table (**Fig. 159 b**). The patient bends the knee of the leg not being tested and places the foot on the table, to prevent exaggerated lumbar lordosis. The examiner stabilizes the hemipelvis on the test side.

[4] [5] [6] Starting position and stabilization are the same as for grade 3 (**Fig. 159 c**).
The examiner applies resistance on the anterior side of the lower leg above the ankle.

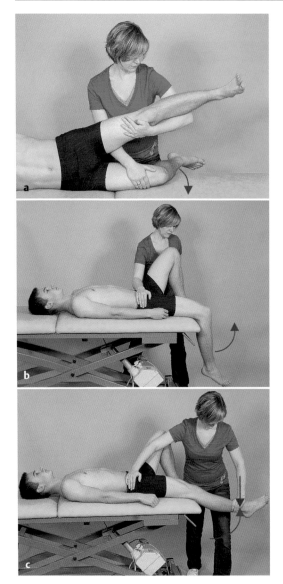

Fig. 159   Testing of knee extension for grades 2, 3, 4, 5, and 6.

■ Flexion at the Knee (Fig. 160)

	Muscle	Origin	Insertion
1	Semimembranosus muscle	Ischial tuberosity	Medial condyle of tibia, joint capsule
2	Semitendinosus muscle	Ischial tuberosity	Superficial pes anserinus (medial condyle of tibia)
	Tibial nerve (L5–S2)		
3	Biceps femoris muscle		
	Long head	Ischial tuberosity	Head of fibula
	Tibial nerve (L5–S2)		
	Short head	Lateral lip of linea aspera, lateral femoral intermuscular septum	Head of fibula
	Common peroneal nerve (S1–S2)		
	Gracilis muscle	Inferior ramus of pubis	Superficial pes anserinus (medial condyle of tibia)
	Obturator nerve (L2–L4)		
	Sartorius muscle	Anterior superior iliac spine	Superficial pes anserinus (medial condyle of tibia)
	Femoral nerve (L1–L3)		
	Gastrocnemius muscle		
	Medial head	Medial condyle of femur	Calcaneal tuberosity
	Lateral head	Lateral condyle of femur	Calcaneal tuberosity
	Tibial nerve (S1–S2)		
	Popliteus muscle	Lateral epicondyle of femur	Posterior surface of tibia
	Tibial nerve (L4–S1)		
	Plantaris muscle	Proximal to lateral condyle of femur, knee joint capsule	Medial border of Achilles tendon
	Tibial nerve (S1–S2)		

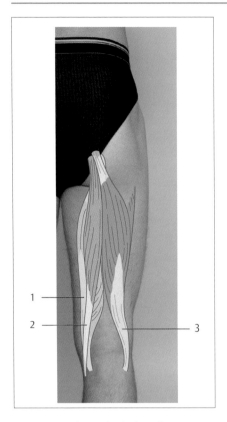

Fig. 160   Muscles involved in knee flexion:
1   Semimembranosus muscle
2   Semitendinosus muscle
3   Biceps femoris muscle

> ## Clinical Symptoms
>
> **Shortening:** The patient is unable to sit with the legs extended while maintaining physiological lordotic lumbar curvature. If the lumbar lordosis is maintained, 70° to 80° hip flexion with the knee joint extended is considered to be a normal range of motion.
>
> However, shortening will not be equally evident on both sides. In this case, the uneven action of the hamstring muscles when the patient is sitting with the legs extended causes the pelvis to twist. This is caused by posterior rotation of the ilium toward the more shortened side. This may result in functional disturbances in the sacro-iliac joints and the lumbar, pelvic, and hip regions.
>
> **Weakness:** If both sides are weakened, pelvic tilt may be present when the patient is standing. Weakness may manifest itself by hyperextension of the knee (see p. 337).

[1] The examiner palpates the muscles, with the patient prone. The semimembranosus, semitendinosus, and biceps femoris muscles can be palpated on the posterior side of the knee joint. The popliteus and plantaris muscles are covered by the gastrocnemius muscles and cannot be palpated.

The following muscles, which participate in knee flexion, will be easier to palpate when they are actively performing their primary action:

- gracilis muscle (hip adduction, see pp. 274 and 275)
- sartorius muscle (hip flexion, see pp. 264 and 265)
- gastrocnemius muscle (ankle plantar flexion, see pp. 300 and 301).

[2] Testing is performed with the patient lying on one side (**Fig. 161 a**). The examiner holds the patient's top leg. The leg being tested is on the bottom and flexed at the hip and knee. The examiner stabilizes the thigh near the knee joint, to prevent compensatory hip flexion.

[3] The patient is prone (**Fig. 161 b**). The examiner stabilizes the pelvis on the side being tested, to prevent the patient from externally rotating and flexing the hip joint.

[4] [5] [6] Starting position and stabilization are the same as for grade 3 (**Fig. 161 c**).

The examiner applies resistance on the posterior side of the lower leg above the ankle joint.

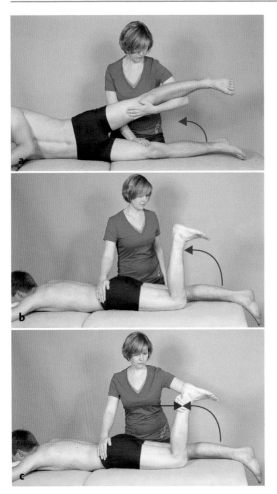

Fig. 161 Testing of knee flexion for grades 2, 3, 4, 5, and 6.

Ankle Joint

■ Dorsiflexion at the Ankle (Fig. 162)

	Muscle	Origin	Insertion
1	*Tibialis anterior muscle*	Lateral surface of tibia, interosseous membrane	Plantar surface of medial cuneiform, first metatarsal
	Deep peroneal nerve (L4–L5)		
2	*Extensor digitorum longus muscle*	Lateral condyle of tibia, head and border of anterior fibula, crural fascia, interosseous membrane	Posterior aponeuroses of second to fifth toes
	Deep peroneal nerve (L5–S1)		
3	*Extensor hallucis longus muscle*	Medial surface of fibula, interosseous membrane	Distal phalanx of first toe
	Deep peroneal nerve (L4–S1)		

Clinical Symptoms

Shortening: Restricted plantar flexion and impaired toe-off. In extreme cases, the patients will develop pes cavus. Shortening of the long toe extensors is described on pages 312 and 320.

Weakness: The patient is unable to adequately lift the distal part of the foot during the swing phase (foot drop). To compensate, the patient increases hip and knee flexion, which results clinically in high stepping (steppage gait pattern) (see p. 339). Balance is impaired when the patient is standing on the affected leg.

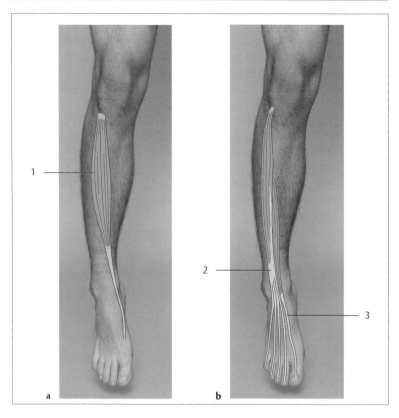

Fig. 162   Muscles involved in dorsiflexion at the ankle joint:
1   Tibialis anterior muscle
2   Extensor digitorum longus muscle
3   Extensor hallucis longus muscle

1⃞ The patient is supine. The knee joint is flexed and the foot hangs off the end of the table, or is positioned so that the heel is not constrained. It is easiest to perform palpation when the patient's lower leg is placed against the examiner's leg.

The tibialis anterior muscle is clearly visible and can be palpated during extension with simultaneous ankle supination.

2⃞ The patient lies on one side (**Fig. 163a**). The patient's foot hangs over the edge of the table. The knee is flexed slightly and the examiner stabilizes the lower leg above the medial malleolus.

3⃞ The patient sits at the edge of the treatment table (**Fig. 163b**). The examiner stabilizes the lower leg above the ankle joint.

4⃞5⃞6⃞ Starting position and stabilization are the same as for grade 3 (**Fig. 163c**).

The examiner applies resistance to the front of the foot.

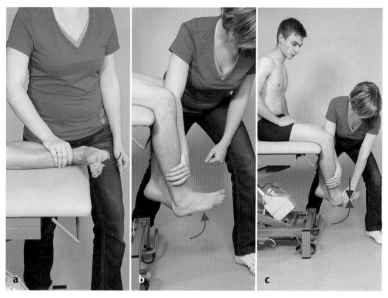

Fig. 163 Testing of ankle dorsiflexion for grades 2, 3, 4, 5, and 6.

■ Plantar Flexion at the Ankle (Fig. 164)

	Muscle	Origin	Insertion
1	*Gastrocnemius muscle*		
	Medial head	Medial condyle of femur	Calcaneal tuberosity
	Lateral head	Lateral condyle of femur	Calcaneal tuberosity
	Tibial nerve (S1–S2)		
2	*Soleus muscle*	Head of fibula, posterior aspect of fibula, soleal line of tibia	Calcaneal tuberosity
	Tibial nerve (S1–S2)		
	Flexor hallucis longus muscle	Posterior aspect of fibula, interosseous membrane, posterior intermuscular septum of leg	Distal phalanx of first toe
	Tibial nerve (S1–S3)		
	Flexor digitorum longus muscle	Posterior aspect of tibia	Distal phalanges of second to fifth toes
	Tibial nerve (S1–S3)		
	Tibialis posterior muscle	Interosseous membrane, posterior aspect of tibia and fibula	Navicular tuberosity, medial, intermediate, and lateral cuneiform
	Tibial nerve (L4–L5)		
	Peroneus longus muscle	Head of fibula, tibiofibular joint, proximal area of fibula	Tuberosity of first metatarsal, medial cuneiform
	Superficial peroneal nerve (L5–S1)		
	Peroneus brevis muscle	Lateral aspect of fibula	Tuberosity of fifth metatarsal
	Superficial peroneal nerve (L5–S1)		
	Plantaris muscle	Lateral condyle of femur, knee joint capsule	Calcaneal tuberosity
	Tibial nerve (S1–S2)		

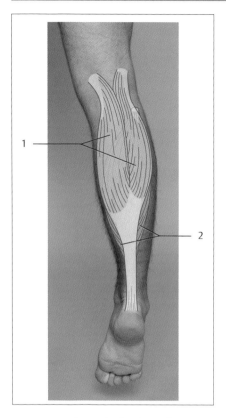

Fig. 164 Muscles involved in plantar flexion at the ankle joint:
1   Gastrocnemius muscle
2   Soleus muscle

Clinical Symptoms

Shortening: Shortening leads to foot drop. Since most plantar flexors also produce supination, the foot will likely also be supinated. The foot drop causes the leg on the affected side to be functionally longer and alters the physiological gait pattern (see pp. 338 and 339).

Weakness: The strength of the toe-off phase is reduced proportionally with the damage. The patient is unable to stand on his or her tiptoes on one leg, and the ability to bounce is significantly diminished. The patient will also develop a claw foot. Since the gastrocnemius muscle is also involved in knee flexion, the knee will tend to be hyperextended. Here too, the patient's balance will be impaired while standing on the affected leg.

[1] For palpation, the patient is prone with the knee slightly flexed. The plantaris muscle is located below the lateral head of the gastrocnemius muscle and cannot be palpated.

The following muscles, which participate in ankle plantar flexion, will be easier to palpate when they are actively performing their primary action:

- flexor hallucis longus muscle (flexion of the big toe, see pp. 324–327)
- flexor digitorum longus muscle (toe flexion, see pp. 316–319)
- tibialis posterior muscle (supination at the subtalar joint, see pp. 304–307)
- pereonus longus and brevis muscles (pronation at the subtalar joint, see pp. 308–311).

[2] The patient is prone, with the knee joint extended and the foot hanging over the edge of the table (**Fig. 165 a**).

The examiner stabilizes the lower leg above the ankle joint. The movement must be performed in the ankle joint and must not be simulated by flexing the toes.

[3] Starting position and stabilization are the same as for evaluation of grade 2 muscle strength (**Fig. 165 b**). The examiner applies maximum resistance to the underside of the foot and heel.

[4] The patient stands on the leg being tested (**Fig. 165 c**). The patient rises up onto tiptoes through the full range of motion.

[5] Starting position is the same as for grade 4. The movement is executed five times.

[6] Starting position is the same as for grade 4. The movement is executed ten times.

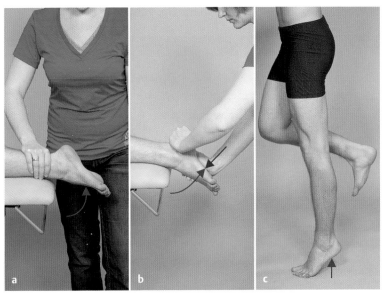

Fig. 165   Testing of plantar flexion at the ankle joint for grades 2, 3, 4, 5, and 6.

■ Supination at the Subtalar Joint (Fig. 166)

	Muscle	Origin	Insertion
1	*Gastrocnemius muscle*		
	Medial head	Medial condyle of femur	Calcaneal tuberosity
	Lateral head	Lateral condyle of femur	Calcaneal tuberosity
	Tibial nerve (S1–S2)		
2	*Soleus muscle*	Head of fibula, posterior third of fibula, soleal line of tibia, tendinous arch of soleus	Calcaneal tuberosity
	Tibial nerve (S1–S2)		
3	*Tibialis posterior muscle*	Interosseous membrane, posterior aspect of tibia and fibula	Navicular tuberosity, medial, intermediate, and lateral cuneiform
	Tibial nerve (L4–L5)		
4	*Tibialis anterior muscle*	Lateral surface of tibia, interosseous membrane, crural fascia	Plantar surface of medial cuneiform, first metatarsal
	Deep peroneal nerve (L4–L5)		
5	*Flexor digitorum longus muscle*	Posterior aspect of tibia	Distal phalanges of second to fifth toes
	Tibial nerve (S1–S3)		
6	*Flexor hallucis longus muscle*	Posterior aspect of fibula, interosseous membrane, posterior intermuscular septum of leg	Distal phalanx of first toe
	Tibial nerve (S1–S3)		
7	*Extensor hallucis longus muscle*	Medial surface of fibula, interosseous membrane	Distal phalanx of first toe
	Deep peroneal nerve (L4–S1)		

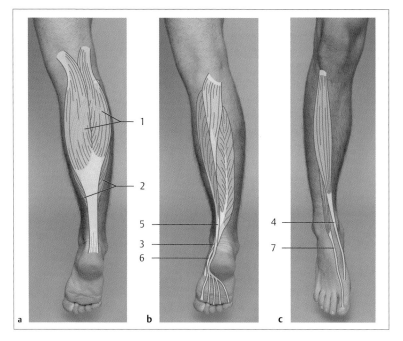

Fig. 166 Muscles involved in subtalar joint supination:

1   Gastrocnemius muscle
2   Soleus muscle
3   Tibialis posterior muscle
4   Tibialis anterior muscle
5   Flexor digitorum longus muscle
6   Flexor hallucis longus muscle
7   Extensor hallucis longus muscle

Clinical Symptoms

Shortening: The foot is inverted (talipes equinovarus). The lateral side of the sole is overloaded when the patient walks. The main load is on the forefoot in the varus position.

Since most of the supinators also produce plantar flexion, refer to the section on shortening during plantar flexion (see p. 301).

Weakness: Depending on the severity of the weakness, the patient will develop talipes equinovalgus. The arch of the foot drops and the medial border of the sole is more heavily loaded. Here too, the patient's balance will be impaired.

☐1 For palpation, the patient is supine with the knee slightly flexed and the foot extended beyond the end of the table. It is easiest to perform palpation when the patient's lower leg is pressed against the examiner's leg. It is easiest to palpate the tibialis posterior muscle when the foot is simultaneously plantar flexed and supinated.

If the examiner is not sure about innervation, all the other muscles involved in supination of the subtalar joint will be easier to test when they are actively performing their primary action:

- gastrocnemius muscle (ankle plantar flexion, see pp. 300 and 301)
- soleus muscle (ankle plantar flexion, see pp. 300 and 301)
- tibialis anterior muscle (ankle dorsiflexion, see pp. 296 and 297)
- flexor digitorum longus muscle (toe joint flexion, see pp. 316 and 317)
- flexor hallucis longus muscle (big toe flexion, see pp. 324 and 325)
- extensor hallucis longus muscle (big toe extension, see pp. 320 and 321)

☐2 The patient is seated, with the legs extended (**Fig. 167 a**). The examiner stabilizes the patient's lower leg above the ankle.

Since most of the supinators also induce plantar flexion, the patient performs the movement in plantar flexion.

☐3 The patient lies on one side, with the foot extended beyond the end of the table (**Fig. 167 b**). The examiner stabilizes the patient's lower leg above the medial malleolus.

☐4 ☐5 ☐6 Starting position and stabilization are the same as for grade 3 (**Fig. 167 c**).

The examiner applies resistance to the first metatarsal.

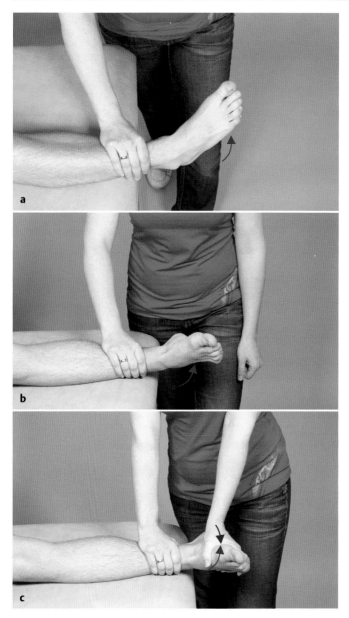

Fig. 167   Testing of subtalar joint supination for grades 2, 3, 4, 5, and 6.

■ Pronation at the Subtalar Joint (Fig. 168)

	Muscle	Origin	Insertion
1	*Peroneus longus muscle* Superficial peroneal nerve (L5–S1)	Head of fibula, capsule of tibiofibular joint, proximal section of fibula	Tuberosity of first metatarsal bone, medial cuneiform
2	*Peroneus brevis muscle* Superficial peroneal nerve (L5–S1)	Lateral aspect of fibula	Tuberosity of fifth metatarsal bone
3	*Extensor digitorum longus muscle* Deep peroneal nerve (L5–S1)	Lateral condyle of tibia, head of fibula, border of anterior fibula, crural fascia, interosseous membrane	Posterior aponeuroses of second to fifth toes

Clinical Symptoms

Shortening: Results in talipes equinovalgus deformity. In this clinical condition, the primary load is on the medial border of the foot during gait.

Weakness: Lateral stability of the subtalar joint is compromised, which can lead to sprains (supination trauma). In patients with this condition, the patient's balance while standing on one leg should also be tested.

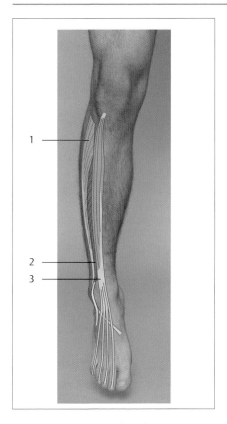

Fig. 168   Muscles involved in subtalar joint pronation:
1   Peroneus longus muscle
2   Peroneus brevis muscle
3   Extensor digitorum longus muscle

1. The patient is supine, with the knee slightly flexed and the foot extended beyond the end of the table. It is easiest to perform palpation when the patient's lower leg is pressed against the examiner's leg.

   It is easier to palpate the extensor digitorum longus muscle when it is performing its primary function (toe joint extension, see pp. 312 and 313).

2. The patient sits with the legs extended and the foot extending beyond the edge of the table (**Fig. 169a**).

3. The patient lies on one side (**Fig. 169b**). The patient's foot extends beyond the end of the table. The examiner stabilizes the patient's lower leg above the lateral malleolus.

4. 5. 6. Starting position and stabilization are the same as for grade 3 (**Fig. 169c**).

   The examiner applies resistance to the fifth metatarsal.

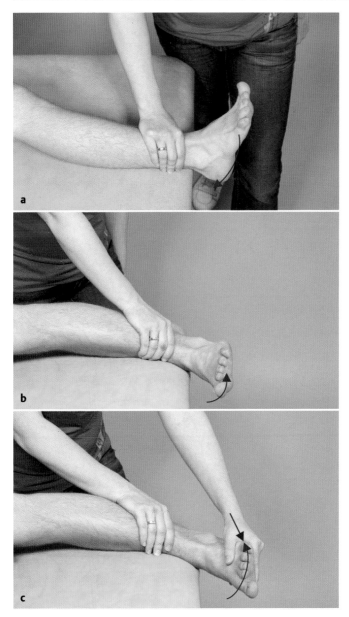

Fig. 169 Testing of subtalar joint pronation for grades 2, 3, 4, 5, and 6.

Toe Joints

■ Extension of the Toes (Fig. 170)

	Muscle	Origin	Insertion
1	*Extensor digitorum longus muscle*	Lateral condyle of tibia, head of fibula, border of anterior fibula, crural fascia, interosseous membrane	Posterior aponeuroses of second to fifth toes
	Deep peroneal nerve (L5–S1)		
2	*Extensor digitorum brevis muscle*	Calcaneus, inferior extensor retinaculum	Posterior aponeuroses of second to fifth toes
	Deep peroneal nerve (S1–S2)		

Clinical Symptoms

Shortening: Development of claw toe deformity.

Weakness: If the extensor digitorum longus muscle is weakened, the reduced strength will tend to manifest itself through slight weakness of the foot dorsiflexors.

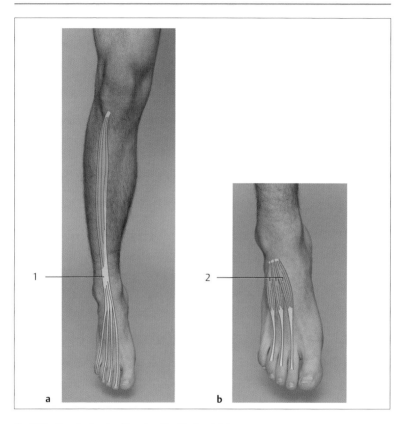

Fig. 170 Muscles involved in extending the toe joints:
1 Extensor digitorum longus muscle
2 Extensor digitorum brevis muscle

1. The examiner palpates these muscles, with the patient sitting with the legs extended. The upper ankle is in a neutral position.
2. The patient sits with the legs extended (**Fig. 171 a**). The examiner stabilizes the forefoot distally at the second to fifth metatarsal bones, near the joint. The movement is executed over a partial range of motion.
3. Starting position and stabilization are the same as for evaluation of grade 2 muscle strength. The movement is executed through the full range of motion.
4. 5. 6. Starting position and stabilization are the same as for grade 2 (**Fig. 171 b**).

The examiner applies resistance to the proximal, medial, and distal phalanges of the toes.

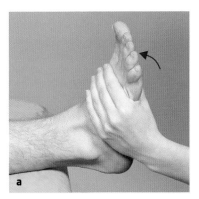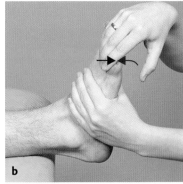

Fig. 171   Testing of toe extension for grades 2, 3, 4, 5, and 6.

■ Flexion of the Toes (Fig. 172)

	Muscle	Origin	Insertion
1	*Flexor digitorum longus muscle* Tibial nerve (S1–S3)	Posterior aspect of tibia	Distal phalanges of second to fifth toes
2	*Flexor digitorum brevis muscle* Medial plantar nerve (L5–S1)	Inferior surface of calcaneal tuberosity, proximal section of plantar aponeurosis	Medial phalanges of second to fifth toes
	Lumbricals Medial plantar nerve (first, second, third lumbricals), lateral plantar nerve (fourth lumbrical) (L5–S2)	Medial sides of individual tendons of long toe flexor	Medial border of proximal phalanges of second to fifth toes, posterior aponeuroses of second to fifth toes
	Dorsal interossei muscles Lateral plantar nerve (S1–S2)	Surfaces of all metatarsals facing each other, long plantar ligament	Bases of the proximal phalanges of second to fourth toes
	Plantar interossei muscles Lateral plantar nerve (S1–S2)	Medial sides of third to fifth metatarsals	Medial sides of bases of proximal phalanges of third to fifth toes
	Flexor digiti minimi brevis muscle Lateral plantar nerve (S1–S2)	Base of fifth metatarsal	Base of proximal phalanx of fifth toe

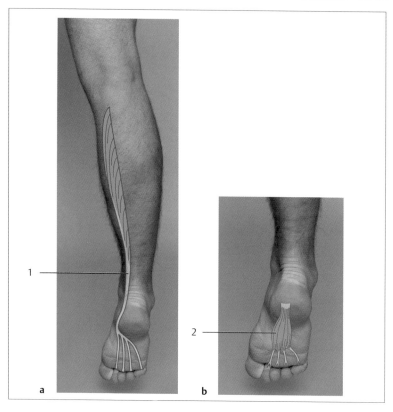

a   b

Fig. 172   Muscles involved in flexing the toe joints:
1   Flexor digitorum longus muscle
2   Flexor digitorum brevis muscle

Clinical Symptoms

Shortening: Flexed position of the toe joints. Disturbances can be apparent during the toe-off phase.

Weakness: Development of claw and hammer toes and flattening of the arch (talipes planus).

1⃣ The examiner palpates the toe flexors, with the patient seated with the legs extended. The ankle joint is in a neutral position. Of the muscles involved in the movement, only the flexor digitorum longus and dorsal interossei muscles can be palpated.

2⃣ The patient sits with the legs extended (**Fig. 173 a**). The examiner stabilizes the forefoot at the distal part of the second to fifth metatarsal bones near the joint. The movement is executed over a partial range of motion.

3⃣ Starting position and stabilization are the same as for evaluation of grade 2 muscle strength. The movement is executed through the full range of motion.

4⃣5⃣6⃣ Starting position and stabilization are the same as for grade 2 (**Fig. 173 b**).
The examiner applies resistance to the proximal, medial, and distal phalanges of the second to fifth toes.

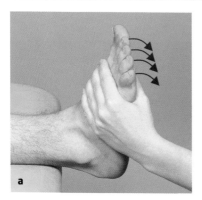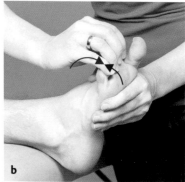

Fig. 173   Testing of toe flexion for grades 2, 3, 4, 5, and 6.

■ Extension of the Big Toe (Hallux) (Fig. 174)

	Muscle	Origin	Insertion
1	*Extensor hallucis longus muscle* Deep peroneal nerve (L4–S1)	Medial surface of fibula, interosseous membrane	Distal phalanx of first toe
2	*Extensor hallucis brevis muscle* Deep peroneal nerve (S1–S2)	Calcaneus	Posterior aponeurosis of first toe

Clinical Symptoms

Shortening: Development of hammer toe. The metatarsophalangeal joint is hyperextended. This, in turn, stretches the flexor hallucis longus muscle and pulls the distal interphalangeal joint into flexion.

Weakness: If the extensor hallucis longus muscle is weakened, the loss of strength will tend to manifest itself through slight weakness of the ankle dorsiflexors.

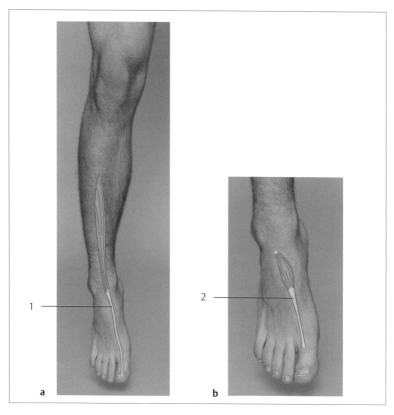

Fig. 174   Muscles that extend the joints of the big toe:
1   Extensor hallucis longus muscle
2   Extensor hallucis brevis muscle

1̄ The examiner palpates these muscles, with the patient sitting with the legs extended. The ankle joint is in a neutral position.

2̄ The patient sits with the legs extended (**Fig. 175 a**). The examiner stabilizes the forefoot at the distal end of the first metatarsal near the joint. The movement is executed over a partial range of motion.

3̄ Starting position and stabilization are the same as for evaluation of grade 2 muscle strength. The movement is executed through the full range of motion.

4̄ 5̄ 6̄ Starting position and stabilization are the same as for grade 2 (**Fig. 175 b**).

The examiner applies resistance to the proximal and distal phalanges of the big toe.

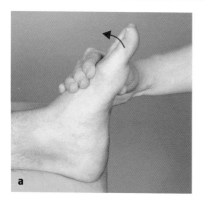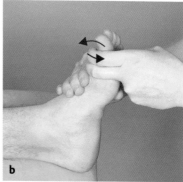

Fig. 175   Testing of extension in the joints of the big toe for grades 2, 3, 4, 5, and 6.

■ Flexion in the Big Toe (Hallux) (Fig. 176)

	Muscle	Origin	Insertion
1	*Flexor hallucis longus muscle* Tibial nerve (S1–S3)	Posterior aspect of fibula, interosseous membrane, posterior intermuscular septum of leg	Base of proximal phalanx of first toe
	Flexor hallucis brevis muscle Medial plantar nerve (L5–S1)	Medial cuneiform, long plantar ligament, tendon of tibialis posterior muscle	Medial and lateral sesamoid bone, proximal phalanx of first toe

Clinical symptoms

Shortening: The big toe is flexed. Depending on the severity, the toe-off phase during walking is disturbed.

Weakness: Weakness of the big toe flexors can result in development of a hammer toe deformity, since the big toe extensors are stronger and pull the big toe joint into hyperextension. The flexor hallucis longus muscle stretched in this way pulls the distal toe joint into flexion. At the same time, weakness in these muscles negatively affects balance.

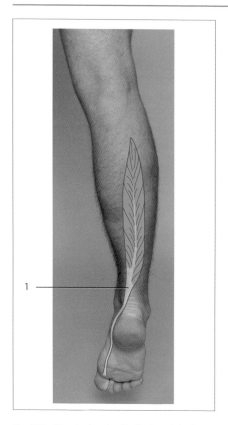

Fig. 176   Muscles involved in flexion of the big toe:
1   Flexor hallucis longus muscle

[1] The examiner palpates the flexors of the big toe, with the patient seated with the legs extended. The ankle joint is in a neutral position. The flexor hallucis brevis muscle cannot be palpated.

[2] The patient sits with the legs extended (**Fig. 177 a**). The examiner stabilizes the forefoot at the distal end of the first metatarsal near the joint. The movement is executed over a partial range of motion.

[3] Starting position and stabilization are the same as for evaluation of grade 2 muscle strength. The movement is executed through the full range of motion.

[4][5][6] Starting position and stabilization are the same as for grade 2 (**Fig. 177 b**).

The examiner applies resistance to the proximal and distal phalanges of the big toe.

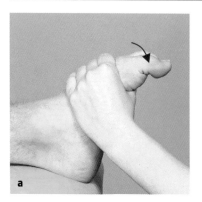 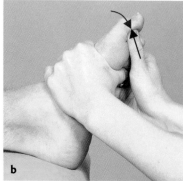

Fig. 177   Testing of flexion in the big toe joints for grades 2, 3, 4, 5, and 6.

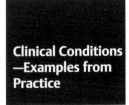

Clinical Conditions —Examples from Practice

This section decribes the most important clinical conditions of the lower extremity that are most commonly observed during testing and therapy.

To better explain deviations from the normal range due to weakness or contractures of the described muscles or muscle functions, the normal physiological condition is described.

In so doing, the foundation for recognizing deviations and influencing them through therapy is provided. Changes in *muscle length* and *muscle strength* cause muscular imbalances. The severity of the disturbed synergy will determine the extent of clinical symptoms.

Even minor deviations over an extended period of time can change static equilibrium. Owing to persistent pathological loading, they can cause damage to all of the joints of the lower extremity, the sacro-iliac joints, and the joints of the entire spinal column, and, in extreme cases, can also damage the joints of the upper extremity.

Weakness of the Hip Extensors

The hip extensors and flexors hold the pelvis of a standing person in unstable equilibrium in the transverse plane. The upper body's line of gravity precisely intersects the flexion–extension axis of the hip joint; both muscle groups have to perform minimal work to keep a person balanced in this position (**Fig. 178**).

If the extensors are weaker, the pelvis will be pulled forward, owing to tension in the flexors, which are stronger. This pelvic tilt results in the center of gravity shifting in front of the flexion–extension axis.

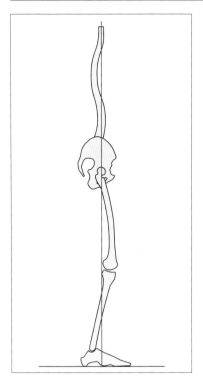

Fig. 178 Normal path of the center of gravity line.

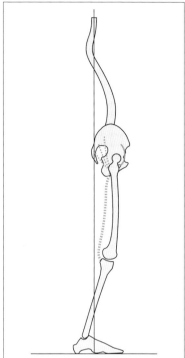

Fig. 179 Backward bending of the upper body to relieve the weakened hip extensors.

Since the patient cannot actively compensate for this shifting, he or she must use passive measures to counteract the traction force of the flexors.

Bending the upper body backward causes the pelvis to passively right itself and in turn hyperextends the hip joints. The upper body's line of gravity is now located behind flexion–extension axis of the hip joint (**Fig. 179**). The muscles of the anterior trunk are hyperactive.

The iliofemoral ligaments prevent the hip joint from going into excessive hyperextension. They prevent the pelvis from tilting too far backward. In so doing, they provide the patient with passive stability, allowing him or her to stand even if the extensors are weak.

Shortening of the Hip Flexors

Flexion of the hip joint can be accomplished in two different ways, depending on which part of the joint is the fixed component and which part is the mobile one.

If the pelvis is the fixed component, flexion is accomplished by raising the leg, for example, the leg swing during walking. If the leg is the fixed component, the patient will flex the hip joint by tilting the pelvis, for example, bending the upper body forward while standing.

A hip flexor contracture therefore causes the pelvis to tilt if the thigh is fixed. The body's line of gravity shifts forward. To counteract this shift, several spontaneous compensatory mechanisms are required: lumbar hyperlordosis, slight knee flexion, and ankle hyperextension (**Fig. 180**).

If the hip flexors are shortened unilaterally, or if shortening is more pronounced on one side, the hemipelvis on the affected side will be tilted forward to a greater extent. In the lower extremity, knee flexion is also used to compensate for contracture on the affected side. Tilting the pelvis and flexing the knee joint functionally shortens the leg, which causes the affected hemipelvis to drop (**Fig. 181**).

Furthermore, the pelvic obliquity results in a scoliotic posture of the spine. During gait, if there is a unilateral hip contracture, the upper body will be bent forward at the end of the stance phase of the affected leg. The hyperextension of the hip joint required in this phase is hampered by the shortened muscles. When the load shifts to the unaffected side, the upper body will return to an upright position. The gait pattern is characterized by the upper body being rocked back and forth (rocking horse gait).

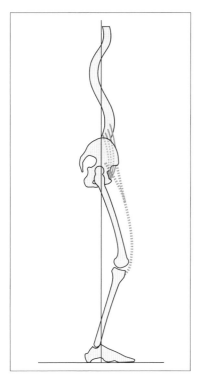

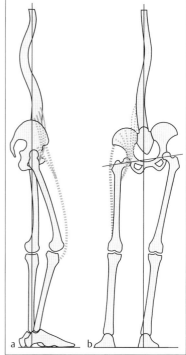

Fig. 180   Bilateral shortening of the hip flexors.

Fig. 181   Unilateral shortening of the hip flexors and its impact on the pelvis and spine.
a Side view.
b Front view.

Shortening of the Hip Abductors and Adductors

Contractures of the hip abductors or adductors always cause the pelvis to shift in the frontal plane. This means that the angles between the load-bearing axes of both legs and a theoretical horizontal line through both hip joints are altered.

This shift causes asymmetrical loading of both legs and results in different pressure in the two sacro-iliac joints, even with minimal shortening. If the shortening is greater, obvious functional differences of leg length will occur. Asymmetrical loading can be determined by having the patient stand on two separate scales.

Hip abductor contracture causes functional leg lengthening, while hip adductor contracture results in functional leg shortening on the affected side. The patient compensates for these differences in leg length by flexing the knee or by abducting the leg on the side that is functionally longer. The entire spinal column will exhibit scoliosis, owing to the resulting pelvic obliquity (**Figs. 182** and **183**).

Weakness of the Hip Abductors

The hip abductors are responsible for stabilizing the pelvis in the frontal plane. This function is clearly evident when the patient stands on one leg, or during the stance phase when walking. In this case, the hip abductors alone are responsible for stabilizing the pelvis in the frontal plane.

During the stance phase, the pelvis tends to tip, owing to the load of the partial body weight (partial body weight is body weight minus standing leg weight) around the center of rotation of the hip joint of the standing leg.

If the pelvis is viewed as a two-arm lever with the hip joint as the center of rotation, the partial body weight (P) and the muscle force (M) of the hip abductors act on the pelvis. This means that the abductors are

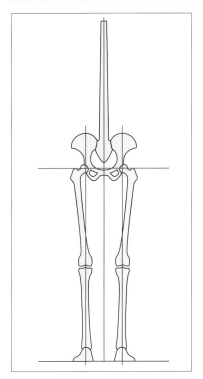

Fig. 182   Trajectory of the line of gravity and the load-bearing axes of the legs if both legs are the same length.

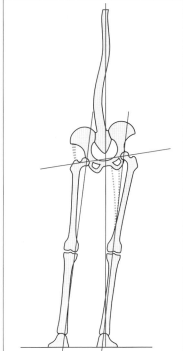

Fig. 183   Trajectory of the line of gravity and the load-bearing axes of the legs if the abductors or adductors are shortened.

strong enough to hold the pelvis horizontal while the patient stands on one leg (**Fig. 184**).

Functional partial paralysis, for instance, after hip surgery, can result in weak abductors (Laube 2009).

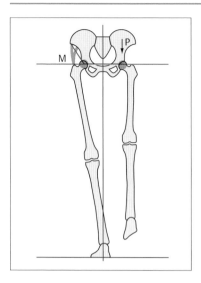

Fig. 184   Stabilization of the pelvis by the hip abductors (M = muscle force, P = partial body weight) when the patient stands on one leg.

If hip abductor strength is reduced, the following compensatory measures can be observed:

- *Trendelenburg sign*: The patient cannot hold partial body weight in the frontal plane during the stance phase of the affected side, and the pelvis tips toward the unaffected side. If there is bilateral abductor insufficiency, a "catwalk gait pattern" can be observed (**Fig. 185**).
- *Duchenne sign*: During the stance phase, the patient attempts to compensate for the lack of strength by shifting the upper body over the pivot point of the hip joint on the affected side. Shifting the body's center of gravity over the pivot point of the hip joint changes the lever arm of the abductors, which can minimize how much force they produce (waddling gait) (**Fig. 186**).

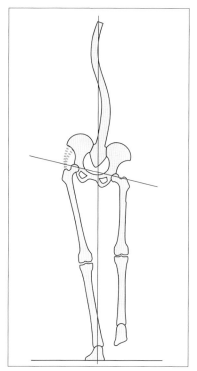

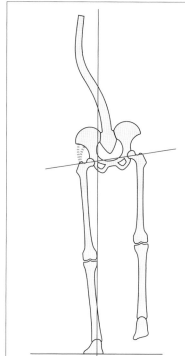

Fig. 185 Trendelenburg sign.

Fig. 186 Duchenne sign.

Weakness of the Quadriceps Femoris Muscle

The quadriceps femoris is a bi-articular muscle. One part of the quadriceps, the rectus femoris muscle, flexes the hip joint. All four parts extend the knee joint. Weakness of the quadriceps femoris muscle manifests itself primarily during knee extension because it is the only active muscle during this movement. During hip flexion, weakness of the quadriceps femoris muscle is less clinically remarkable because other muscles are able to compensate for any lack of strength.

For this reason, deficient knee extension is described next.

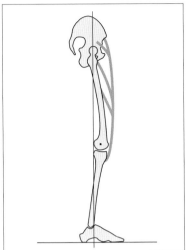 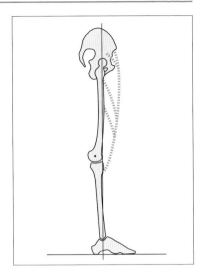

Fig. 187   Trajectory of the loading axis if the quadriceps femoris muscle has normal strength.

Fig. 188   Trajectory of the loading axis if the quadriceps femoris muscle is weakened.

To better understand stabilization of the knee joint, the trajectory of the body's line of gravity relative to the flexion and extension axis of the knee joint must be described first. As soon as the knee joint starts to flex, the line of gravity will shift behind the axis of motion and the quadriceps femoris muscle becomes active to provide stability (**Fig. 187**). If the knee joint is hyperextended, the line of gravity will be in front of the axis of motion and the posterior capsuloligamentous structures will take over stabilizing the knee joint without involvement of the quadriceps femoris muscle (**Fig. 188**).

The patient can shift the line of gravity in front of the axis of motion by tilting the pelvis to bring the upper body forward. The patient uses this compensatory mechanism to passively stabilize the knee joint in extension if the quadriceps femoris muscle is weakened. During gait, hyperextension is increased during the loading phase, since the entire body weight rests on one leg. Functional partial paralysis of the quadriceps femoris muscle is observed as a complication of knee surgery (Laube 2009).

Everyday movements, such as climbing stairs, getting up from a sitting position, or squatting are difficult for the patient or cannot be executed without assistance.

Weakness of the Hamstring Muscles

With the exception of the short head of the biceps femoris muscle, the hamstring muscles act in a bi-articular fashion, flexing the knee and extending the hip. If they are weakened, both functions will be impaired.

When the patient stands upright, and during normal gait, the hamstring muscles extend the hip, for the most part without any assistance from the gluteus maximus muscle. As the strongest knee flexors, they are active posterior stabilizers of the knee joint. When the patient is standing, weakness of the hamstring muscles also manifests itself through increased tilt of the pelvis, owing to the weakened hip extensors, and by hyperextension in the knee joint, owing to the lack of posterior muscular stability.

The clinical presentation when the patient is standing resembles that of weakness of the quadriceps femoris muscle. If the quadriceps is weak, however, hip flexion will still be actively performed to shift the loading axis and hyperextend the knee.

During gait, increased knee hyperextension during the stance phase can be observed if the hamstring muscles are weakened, since the body weight now rests on one leg.

Shortening of the Triceps Surae Muscle

As the name suggests, the triceps surae is composed of three muscle heads: the lateral and medial heads of the gastrocnemius, along with the soleus muscle. They insert together as the Achilles tendon at the calcaneal tuberosity, and produce plantar flexion in the ankle joint and supination in the subtalar joint. In addition to the triceps surae muscle, the plantaris muscle has the same function and can also be shortened.

The heads of the gastrocnemius muscle arise from the medial and lateral femoral condyles and therefore also produce knee flexion.

This function is less important to the strength of knee flexion. However, the gastrocnemius is a muscle that limits knee hyperextension during extension of the ankle joint. Its action in the ankle joint also depends on the amount of knee flexion. When the knee is extended, the muscle has already been stretched and can completely unleash its strength. When the knee is flexed, the muscle is shortened and loses its ability to produce plantar flexion.

Shortening of the triceps surae muscle leads to increased ankle plantar flexion and subtalar supination, which is referred to as foot drop. When standing, the patient compensates for the ensuing functional leg lengthening by flexing the knee (**Fig. 189**).

During gait, the stance phase of the affected leg begins with forefoot contact. The heel does not touch the ground. Knee flexion is maintained during the shortened stance phase. In the swing phase, the leg has to be flexed more at the knee and hip so that the functionally longer leg can swing through. Shortening of the triceps surae muscle frequently occurs after rupture of the Achilles tendon.

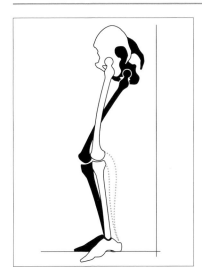

Fig. 189 Shortening of the triceps surae muscle with foot drop position (shown in white). The patient can flex the knee to achieve relative muscle lengthening and, in turn, full extension in the ankle joint (shown in black).

Weakness of the Ankle Dorsiflexors

During normal gait, after the toe-off phase of the leg swing, the forefoot comes off the ground. The patient initiates this lift-off phase by extending the toes and dorsiflexing the ankle joint.

If the ankle dorsiflexors are weakened or paralyzed, the patient can compensate for the absent dorsiflexion by increasing hip and knee flexion. This means that the patient must lift the leg higher during the swing phase to lift the forefoot off the ground. In the subsequent stance phase, contact with the ground does not begin with the heel, as usual, but with the tip of the foot that is hanging down. This gait, characterized by loss of the foot dorsiflexors, is referred to as *steppage* gait or *high stepping* (**Figs. 190** and **191**).

Weakness of the foot dorsiflexors is often caused by a herniated disk, or anterior compartment syndrome of the lower leg.

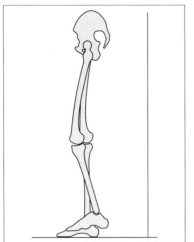

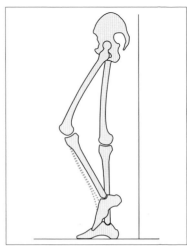

Fig. 190   Normal gait pattern.

Fig. 191   Increased hip and knee flexion, owing to weakness of the ankle dorsiflexors.

7
Questions

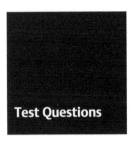

Test Questions

1. Define strength grades 0–6.

2. Name the key muscles for segments C6, C7, L4, and S1.

3. What role do mover muscles play and what role do stabilizer muscles play?

4. What are the symptoms of weak hip extensors?

5. What happens when the hip flexors are shortened?

6. Describe the functional difference in leg length when there is hip abductor and adductor contracture.

7. Describe the limping mechanisms that can occur if the hip abductors are weakened.

8. What do quadriceps femoris muscle weakness and hamstring muscle weakness have in common?

9. Describe the signs of weak ankle dorsiflexors.

10. What is the trajectory of the line of gravity in a person who is standing upright?

11. Which muscles running toward the head play a major role in tilting the pelvis and which ones play a key role in straightening the pelvis?

12. Which muscles are able to lift the thorax?

13. Which three nerves can cause winged scapula if they are damaged?

14. What are the differences between the three types of winged scapula?

15. Which muscles are affected in a patient with Erb palsy?

16. Which muscles are affected in a patient with Klumpke paralysis?

17. Which muscles are paralyzed in a patient with suprascapular nerve palsy?

18. Name the muscles paralyzed due to axillary nerve palsy. Which movements are particularly weakened in this case?

19. Name the muscles affected by musculocutaneous nerve palsy.

20. Describe the typical clinical presentation of radial nerve palsy, ulnar nerve palsy, and median nerve palsy.

21. What is the positive bottle sign and what causes it?

22. How do muscle tone and monosynaptic reflex activity change in cases of central and peripheral nervous system disturbances?

23. In a patient with a herniated disk, why is testing for tactile sensation less reliable than testing for pain sensation?

24. Which symptoms are exhibited in a patient with disk herniation at L4–L5 when key muscles, sensory perception, and monosynaptic reflexes are tested?

25. Which movement components are involved in thumb opposition and reposition?

26. Which movements of the shoulder joint is the deltoid muscle involved in?

27. Which shoulder movements may be limited if the teres major muscle is shortened?

28. How does shortening of the pectoralis minor muscle affect the position of the shoulder and which shoulder movements will be limited?

29. Which hip movements may be limited if the tensor of fascia lata muscle is shortened?

30. Which segment is affected if the C5–C6 disk is herniated and which one is affected if the L4–L5 disk is herniated?

31. Which monosynaptic reflex should be tested if the C5–C6 disk is herniated and which one should be tested if the L4–L5 disk is herniated?

32. What can be triggered by weak supinators of the subtalar joint?

33. What symptom may occur if the pronators of the subtalar joint are weak?

34. Which muscles must be tested if the shoulder cannot be elevated with full strength?

35. What are the symptoms of weak wrist flexors?

36. Is poliomyelitis a central or peripheral nervous system disorder?

37. Do patients with poliomyelitis have sensory impairment?

38. Name the causes of root compression.

39. What are the symptoms of polyneuropathy?

40. Name the symptoms of central spastic paresis.

41. Name the symptoms of peripheral flaccid paralysis.

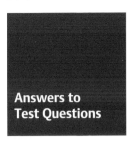

Answers to Test Questions

1. 0 = No visible or palpable contraction of a muscle involved in the movement.
   1 = Visible or palpable contraction of a muscle involved in the movement.
   2 = The muscle can complete the full range of motion when the force of gravity is minimized.
   3 = The muscle can complete the full range of motion against the resistance of gravity.
   4 = The muscle can complete the full range of motion against the resistance of gravity and against moderate resistance.
   5 = The muscle can complete the full range of motion against the resistance of gravity and against maximum resistance.
   6 = The muscle can complete the full range of motion against the resistance of gravity and against maximum resistance and can perform the movement at least 10 times.

2. C6 Extensor carpi radialis longus and brevis muscles
   C7 Triceps brachii muscle
   L4 Tibialis anterior muscle
   S1 Triceps surae muscle

3. Mover muscles maintain a certain plane during a movement. They intervene to correct the movement during flexion or extension, for example, through rotation, abduction, or adduction. Stabilizer muscles are muscles that attach the scapula to the trunk, or that attach the pelvis to the trunk. The stabilizer muscles hold one body part immobile while another body part is moving.

4. To counteract the stronger hip flexors and avoid pelvic tilt, the patient bends the upper body backward. By doing so, the hip hyperextends, which provides passive stability via the iliofemoral ligaments.

5. Bilateral shortening of the hip flexors is characterized by increased pelvic tilt with the upper body bent forward, as well as limited hip extension, lumbar hyperlordosis, knee flexion to compensate for the shift of the upper body, and increased extension in the ankle joints. In unilateral shortening of the hip flexors, the hemipelvis on the affected side is turned forward and the knee joint is flexed. The unilateral shortening leads to functional leg shortening on the affected side, as well as to pelvic obliquity and scoliotic posture of the spine.

6. Contracture of the abductors causes functional leg lengthening on the affected side; shortening of the adductors causes functional leg shortening on the affected side.

7. *Duchenne sign*: during the stance phase of the weakened side, the patient shifts the upper body over the affected hip to relieve the muscles. *Trendelenburg sign*: during the stance phase of the affected side, the opposite hemipelvis tips downward, since the abductors are unable to hold the pelvis.

8. Hyperextension of the knee, as well as passive stability via the posterior capsuloligamentous structures.

9. The lack of extension in the ankle joint requires increased hip and knee flexion to lift the forefoot off the ground. The first contact with the ground in the incipient stance phase of the affected side is with the forefoot.

10. Viewed from the side, the line of gravity runs from the external auditory canal to the hip joint, through the center of the knee joint, and meets the foot at the navicular bone.

11. Pelvic tilting is primarily controlled by the hip flexors and pelvic straightening is controlled by the hip extensors.

12. The erector trunci, scalene, sternocleidomastoid, pectoralis major, and pectoralis minor muscles in interaction with the scapula fixators.

13. Accessory nerve—trapezius muscle
    Long thoracic nerve—anterior serratus muscle
    Dorsal scapular nerve—rhomboid muscles

14. If the accessory nerve is damaged, the scapula clearly moves medially. If the long thoracic nerve is damaged, the scapula is pulled medially. If the dorsal scapular nerve is affected, the scapula moves only slightly laterally. Winged scapula and weakness when lifting the arm are not as evident as in the other two forms.

15. The deltoid, teres major, supraspinatus, infraspinatus, anterior serratus, rhomboid, biceps brachii, brachioradialis, and supinator muscles are affected.

16. The finger flexors, lumbricals, and interossei muscles are affected.

17. The supraspinatus and infraspinatus muscles are paralyzed.

18. The deltoid and teres minor muscles are paralyzed. Forward flexion, abduction, and external rotation at the shoulder joint are weakened.

19. The strength of the biceps brachii, brachialis, and coracobrachialis muscles is reduced.

20. Radial nerve palsy—wrist drop
    Median nerve palsy—ape hand
    Ulnar nerve palsy—claw hand

21. The positive bottle sign occurs when the muscles at the base of the thumb are lost, owing to median nerve palsy. When the patient attempts to grasp a bottle with the affected hand, he or she will be unable to sufficiently abduct the thumb; as a consequence, the web between the thumb and index finger does not touch the bottle.

22. In central nerve damage, muscle tone and monosynaptic reflex activity are usually increased; in peripheral nerve damage, they are always diminished.

23. There is a high degree of overlap among the dermatomes with regard to tactile sensation, which is not the case for pain sensation.

24. Key muscles: tibialis anterior muscle weakened, quadriceps femoris muscle weakened.
Sensory perception: disturbances in the area of the lateral thigh, lower half of the patella, and medial lower leg down to the medial border of the foot.
Monosynaptic reflexes: knee-jerk reflex weakened.

25. Thumb opposition:
    - Abduction and flexion in the thumb carpometacarpal joint.
    - Flexion in the thumb metacarpophalangeal and interphalangeal joints.

    Thumb reposition:
    - Abduction and extension in the carpometacarpal joint of the thumb.
    - Extension in the thumb metacarpophalangeal and interphalangeal joints.

26. The deltoid muscle is involved in all movements of the shoulder joint.

27. If the teres major muscle is shortened, forward flexion, external rotation, and abduction may be limited.

28. Shortening of the pectoralis minor muscle affects scapular abduction (protraction), which can limit forward flexion, external rotation, and abduction of the arm.

29. Hip extension and adduction may be limited; external rotation may be slightly limited.

30. If the C5–C6 disk is herniated, the C6 segment is affected. If the L4–L5 disk is herniated, segment L4 is affected.

31. If the C5–C6 disk is herniated, the brachioradialis reflex must be tested. If the L4–L5 disk is herniated, the knee-jerk reflex must be tested.

32. Weakness of the ankle joint supinators can bring about talipes valgus.

33. Since the ankle pronators are weak, the foot has insufficient lateral stability, which can lead to a sprain.

34. If forward flexion cannot be performed with full strength, the muscles of the shoulder joint (deltoid, biceps brachii, pectoralis major, coracobrachialis, and supraspinatus muscles) must be tested, along with the muscles that stabilize and move the scapula (trapezius and serratus anterior muscles).

35. When the patient lifts heavy objects with the forearm supinated, he or she cannot hold the wrist in a neutral position. It tips backward.

36. Poliomyelitis affects the peripheral nervous system. Damage affects the anterior horn motor neuron, starting from the synaptic contacts between the first and second motor neuron.

37. Since poliomyelitis consists of inflammation in the area of the anterior horn motor neuron, sensory perception is not disturbed.

38. Herniated disk; degenerative processes in the area of the articular processes.

39. Deficits that are usually bilateral and tend to occur in the distal parts of the extremities. Motor, sensory and autonomic deficits affecting several nerves. Stocking glove sensory loss, flaccid paralysis with considerable muscle atrophy, and trophic skin lesions. Proprioception is also affected; the patient is unsteady when standing and walking.

40. Diminished strength with disturbed fine motor function, increased muscle tone, increased reflex activity, pathological reflexes, diminished or absent monosynaptic reflexes, no degenerative muscle atrophy.

41. Reduced strength or complete loss of strength, reduced muscle tone, diminished or absent muscle reflexes, muscle atrophy.

Bibliography

Benninghoff, A., Goertler, K.: Lehrbuch der Anatomie des Menschen, Bd. 1, 9. Aufl. Urban & Schwarzenberg, München 1964

Brinckmann P., Frobin W., Leivseth G.: Musculoskeletal Biomechanics. Thieme, Stuttgart 2002

Bruegger, A.: Die Erkrankungen des Bewegungsapparates und seines Nervensystems, 2. Aufl. Fischer, Stuttgart 1980

Buckup, K.: Clinical Tests for the Musculoskeletal System. Examinations – Signs – Phenomena, 2nd ed. Thieme, Stuttgart 2008

Daniels, Worthingham: Muskelfunktionsprüfung, 4. Aufl. Fischer, Stuttgart 1982

Dauber, W.: Pocket Atlas of Human Anatomy, Founded by Heinz Feneis, 5th ed. Thieme, Stuttgart 2006

Duus, P.: Duus' Topical Diagnosis in Neurology, 5th ed. Thieme, Stuttgart 2012

Frisch, H.: Programmierte Untersuchung des Bewegungsapparates, 1. Aufl. Springer, Berlin 1983

Gustavsen, R., Streeck R.: Trainingstherapie im Rahmen der Manuellen Medizin, 2. Aufl. Thieme, Stuttgart 1991

Hislop, H.J., Montgomery, J.: Daniels' und Worthinghams Muskeltests. Elsevier, München 1999

Hoppenfeld, S.: Orthopädische Neurologie. Enke, Stuttgart 1980

Janda V.: Manuelle Funktionsdiagnostik, 4. Aufl. Urban & Fischer bei Elsevier, München 2009

Kahle, W.: Color Atlas of Human Anatomy, Vol 3, Nervous System and Sensory Organs, 6th ed. Thieme, Stuttgart, 2010

Kapandji, I.A.: Funktionelle Anatomie der Gelenke, Bd. 1: Obere Extremität, 1984, Bd. 2: Untere Extremität, 1985, Bd. 3: Rumpf und Wirbelsäule. Enke, Stuttgart 1985

Kendall, H.O., Kendall, F.P., Wadsworth, G.E.: Muscles, Testing and Function, 2nd ed. Williams & Wilkins, Baltimore 1971

Klein-Vogelbach, S.: Funktionelle Bewegungslehre, 2. Aufl. Springer, Berlin 1977

von Lanz, T., Wachsmuth W.: Praktische Anatomie, Bd. 1/3: Arm, Bd. 1/4: Bein und Statik. Springer, Berlin 1972

Laube, W.: Sensomotorisches System. Thieme, Stuttgart 2009

Lewitt, K.: Manuelle Medizin, 2. Aufl. J. Barth, Leipzig 1977

Matthiass, H.H.: Klinische Meßmethoden an der Wirbelsäule. In Junghanns H. (Hrsg.), Diagnostik der Wirbelsäulenerkrankungen, Die Wirbelsäule in Forschung und Praxis, Bd. 83. Hippokrates, Stuttgart 1979: 23–29

Meinecke, F.-W.: Verletzungen der Wirbelsäule und des Rückenmarks – spezielle Chirurgie für die Praxis. Thieme, Stuttgart 1980

Montgomery J., Hislop H.J.: Daniel's und Worthingham's Muskeltests: Manuelle Untersuchungstechniken, 8. Aufl. Urban & Fischer bei Elsevier, München 2007

Mumenthaler, M., Mattle H.: Neurology, 4th ed. Thieme, Stuttgart 2003

Pernkopf, E.: Atlas der topografischen und angewandten Anatomie des Menschen, Bd. 1 u. 2, 2. Aufl. Urban & Schwarzenberg, München 1980

Platzer, W.: Color Atlas of Human Anatomy, Vol 1, Locomotor System, 7th ed. Thieme, Stuttgart 2014

Rohen, J.W.: Funktionelle Neuroanatomie Lehrbuch und Atlas, 6. Aufl. Schattauer, Stuttgart 2001

Schmidtbleicher, D.: Zum Problem der Definition des Begriffs Kraftausdauer. In Carl, K., Starischka, S., Stork, H. (Hrsg.), Kraftausdauertraining, Bericht zum BISP-Symposium, Sport und Buch, Köln 1989: 10–30

Schünke, M., Schulte, E., Schumacher, U.: THIEME Atlas of Anatomy Image Collection—Head and Neuroanatomy. Thieme, Stuttgart 2007

Sobotta, J., Becher H.: Atlas der Anatomie des Menschen, Bd. 1 u. 3, 17. Aufl. Urban & Schwarzenberg, München 1972

Tittel, K.: Beschreibende und funktionelle Anatomie des Menschen, 8. Aufl. Fischer, Stuttgart 1978

Winkel, D., Vleeming, A., Fisher, S., Meijer, O.G., Vroege C.: Nichtoperative Orthopädie, Teil 1: Anatomie in vivo; Teil 2: Diagnostik. Fischer, Stuttgart 1985

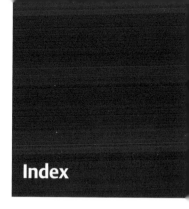

Index

Page numbers in *italics* refer to illustration